Striving

for

Imprefection

per

SCOTT "Q" MARCUS

THINspirational Columnist and Recovering Perfectionist

additional
52^Inspirational
Playful Columns
on Living Well,
Changing Habits,
and Other Acts of Faith

Striving for Imperfection
Volume 2
2nd printing

©2008, 2011 by
Scott Marcus

ISBN: 978-1466436015

Printed in the United States of America

For additional copies of this book, or to hire Scott "Q" Marcus for speaking,
training, consulting or workshops, call 707.442.6243
or scottq@scottqmarcus.com.

To get past what holds you or your business back,
go to www.ThisTimeIMeanIt.com
or
or www.ScottQMarcus.com

02.12.12

To anyone who was ever told:

"You're too fat!"

"You're too skinny."

"You're too stupid."

"You're too much of a nerd."

"You're too old."

"You're too young."

"You'll never make it."

"You don't deserve it."

"You worry too much."

"You don't care enough."

...to anyone who ever doubted.

Yes you can.

Believe.

TABLE OF CONTENTS

Striving

for

Imprefection

per

SCOTT "Q" MARCUS

THINspirational Columnist and Recovering Perfectionist

additional
52^Inspirational
Playful Columns
on Living Well,
Changing Habits,
and Other Acts of Faith

THE RESOLUTION

"I resolve this will be my healthiest year ever!"

"Great! How are you doing that?"

"I start at 4:30 each morning. I bought one of those way cool Zen clocks to gently ease me awake. Then I meditate for 30 minutes. I don't eat unconsciously if I start my day centered and balanced."

"I hear you. No one likes a crooked diet."

"Are you making fun of me?"

"No, just playing; I admire your dedication. What's next?"

"Exercise. I bought top-of-the-line brand name running clothes — $175 for the shoes alone. I also plunked down cash for microfiber rainproof pants, a fleece pullover, and pedometer. You should see it; it counts steps, distance, even calories. So, I do a rigorous warm up followed by a three-mile run and power walk, and end with a cool-down stretch. I have DVDs and a CD to guide me."

"Wow, I'm exhausted just listening."

"There's more. After an aromatherapy shower using four all-natural astringents and a limited design anti-cellulite luffa, I plan meals. I purchased an entire collection of healthy-eating cookbooks, and subscribe to an on-line service that each day provides a new prepare-from-scratch, all-organic recipe tailored to my personal history — which I mix and cook in specially treated cookware."

"Specially treated? How's that?"

"I'm a little fuzzy on the details. But the infomercial said they have 'an exclusive adipose reduction coating that the diet companies don't want us to know about.' They wouldn't lie in their own ads, would they?"

"Heaven forbid! No!"

"Success involves conscious thought. So I write things down. I got a journal for my thoughts and feelings, another for logging exercise, and a third to record calories, fat, fiber, portion sizes, and of course, my weight and measurements."

"Let me guess; you bought a scale too."

CHOICES

I am a "Guy."

In built with "guys," are certain behaviours. For example, I cannot imagine, ever in my wildest dreams, that I would — by choice — use a duvet cover. My wife, conversely, is a dutiful dedicated devotee of the duvet cover.

Of course, truth be known, I would probably not use a topsheet either, opting to merely crawl into bed on top of the bottom sheet and slide snugly under the blankets. Blankets are for cover and warmth. Sheets are for — well, I'm not sure what sheets are for, but they seem appropriate. A topsheet is redundant, especially when it is used with a duvet cover, because the blanket gets more covering than me — which I find illogical and insulting.

I am not a cretin; I do possess a modicum of respectability, and would still use pillowcases. (Alas, I would probably not wash them weekly as my wife prefers.)

As stated, I am, after all, a "Guy."

This column is not a diatribe about the differences between "guys" and "civilized society." I employ the above merely to illustrate the point that there is diversity in what people want. As referenced by Sly Stone, "Different strokes for different folks."

At my weight loss group, we engaged in heavy discussion (um, maybe "intense discussion" would be a better choice of words) lamenting that there is no "Holy Grail of Diets." This "Ultimate Plan" would be known by its specific menu of prescribed (flavorful) foods; an easy, low-intensity, specific, exercise regime; and a predetermined known-in-advance end date. At its conclusion, all excess poundage would have vanished, unhealthy desires evaporated, and self-esteem skyrocketed. We would simply enter the path and arrive complete at the foreseen finish.

Regrettably, losing weight is not so formulaic. One cannot merely eat two ounces of fish, drink four glasses of water, walk three miles, and — "ta da" — be thin. Habit change requires an unending string of adjustments to life's agenda: we must make choices. For some, choice is a low carb thing (although I can't imagine why). For others, it's a "dietary program." Certain people opt for "I'll do it tomorrow." All equally fair choices.

Choice is always an option — and so are its consequences. Choose well.

(But let someone else make the bed.)

DINING WITH THIN FRIENDS

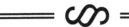

They are among us. Although they seem to be our friends, they are born of out-worldly pods, as they can voraciously, and without regard, consume anything remaining stationary long enough to be pierced by a fork — and not gain an ounce. Be watchful, and you too shall come across them.

I share this recent restaurant encounter:

ME (after a prolonged, stressful, internal dialog between stomach and brain): "I'll have the salad, fat free dressing — on the side. No croutons or cheese."

WAITER: "Would you like anything else?"

ME (sighing): "Yes, a great many things, mostly sweet and fried; but I shall resist yet again as part of the unending torture of trying to knock off the same lousy few pounds. And please take away the basket of bread rolls."

WAITER (addressing Disgustingly Thin Friend Of Mine): "What will you have sir?"

DTFOM (reclaiming the rolls and dipping them in oil): "The BCGE."

WAITER: "Ah, the bucket of cholesterol and grease extravaganza, excellent. Extra butter and melted cheese?"

DTFOM: "Of course. I'd also like the city-size order of fries, egg roll platter, and double onion rings."

Both are drawn to look at me as the sound of my forehead banging a slow, pathetic, rhythmic cadence on the table has attracted attention.

DTFOM (to waiter): "I'd also like a supreme-double-vanilla-mocha-deluxe, extra sugar and whipped cream; and the 'Death by Chocolate' four-pound, six-layer, ice cream and cookie cake, family reunion size."

Upon return, the waiter piles 36 platters of food on the table. To do so requires a rolling serving platter, stand-up folding tray, and three burley assistants. Finally, he squeezes out a miserly few square inches and places down my platter of "rabbit food." (If I seem bitter, I can assure you it only happens during periods of low blood sugar.)

WAITER: "Anything else gentlemen?"

DTFOM: "Not now. But come back, I might still be hungry." As the waiter departs, DTFOM reminds me to close my chops, the slack-jaw appearance is unappealing.

DTFOM smothers his servings with spices, sauces, and sugars. I finish my miserly smattering of wilted lettuce, two cucumber slices, and a cherry tomato, before his first bite. With stomach growling, and inner child on full-throttle cranky, I succumb to my desires and lightly request, "Would you mind if I had a French fry?"

"Not at all," he replies, "but what about your diet?"

ONE OF THESE DAYS

One of these days, I'm going to get back on track with my diet. Really. I'll burst out of bed inspired, invigorated, and enthused. I'll clear the kitchen, throw out the junk food, pull out my motivational books, and start weighing, measuring, and monitoring anything that crosses my lips. No crumb of cuisine will be too trivial to escape my scrutiny. Yep, that's the way you lose weight you know. One of these days, boy am I going to get my eating act together! I'm just so busy right now.

Someday soon I've got to start exercising. I could wake up earlier, strap on some tunes, and stroll around the block. It's just so warm in bed, and I've been waiting for the rain to stop; my raincoat is so old, I'd look silly walking around town in it. I'm looking forward to a patch of blue sky so I can get back out there.

Just as soon as I can get around to it, I need to start a journal. I've been organizing my thoughts — even thinking about jotting down a few notes. I considered using a yellow-lined pad, but I really want to keep my thoughts and feelings for years. Recording something so important on any old bland notebook would be tacky, so I'm toying with buying a deluxe, leather-bound journal — maybe even an expensive pen. When I can put away a few dollars, I'm so there.

In a little while, I think I'll even go again to my meetings. It's just, well, you know how it is: holidays, travel, celebrations... who can control themselves with goodies everywhere? A slip-up here, some sloppiness there — boom — eight pounds! I almost went back last week, except it's so embarrassing to keep putting on the same pounds — so I'll knock them off first, and then head back. In a few weeks, it'll be a better time anyway.

One of these days real soon, I'll get it all together. I've been planning it a long time; I just want to make sure I do it right, no mess-ups allowed. So I'm waiting until life settles down before I get started. Let me tell you though, when the time is perfect, there's no stopping me.

I can feel it coming, one of these days, real soon, right about the corner...

Uncomfortable moments

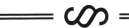

I pride myself on a positive attitude (more times than not). Of course, there are those "nots" when I scratch my graying head of hair in perplexed, somewhat sad, (admittedly slightly judgmental) stupefaction. My soapbox is becoming well worn, so I tried to resist the urge to hoist myself upon it. Alas, 'twas in vain…

The next in a long lineage of supposed godsends for obesity is an over-the-counter fat-blocking pill which prevents 25 percent of the fat one ingests from being absorbed, resulting in weight loss. In studies, obese patients lost about 5-10 pounds more per year (sic) than those who took a placebo. (Of course, those who took a regular walk dropped about 25 pounds — and saved enough cash to buy a thinner wardrobe.)

Hold back the extra-cheesy nachos; there is a dark side.

Since ingested fat must go somewhere, it slides though the digestive track and exits, resulting in a series of rather uncivilized, descriptive, side effects better left unprinted. The less offensive results include a "predisposition toward flatulence" and something euphemistically referred to as "seepage." (I shall not be insulted if you choose to bleach that image from your brain; just writing it makes me cringe.)

Here's my problem: habit change is not fun or easy. On the contrary, it is usually forced upon us, the result of fear or pain. As illustration, I lost 70 pounds because the fear of a future heart attack became more powerful than the comfort of my eating habits. Others quit drinking or stop smoking because reality strikes: stop or die. It is cold, stark truth; from denial's death arises change.

I shan't deny habit change is demanding; anything worth achieving requires some exertion. I also identify with self-doubt as a constant companion. But we disregard that we are simply astonishing creatures, capable of mind-blowing achievements. With focus, we are surely capable of taking a periodic walk, or pushing ourselves away from the table five minutes earlier. I fear we are descending to a low point where it is expected that everything is delivered without effort, therefore sacrificing the exhilaration of accomplishment.

No argument, lifestyle changes can be just plain uncomfortable. But I would think less so than those awkward, embarrassing moments apologizing in public, "Oops, excuse me, I'm taking a weight loss medicine."

I GIVE UP

This will be my final column, because between you, me, and the lamppost, I've had it with dieting.

I have reached my limit of getting on the scale — that obsessive, compulsive, weekly monitoring to determine whether I've put on four ounces or lost seven. I can do without the gnawing in the pit of my stomach each time I stand on that double-dealing, lifeless, white platform with the hellish red flashing LED that screams out my weight. Goodbye weigh-in!

I've just had it with counting calories — forever monitoring nutrition labels, analyzing "saturated" versus "trans fat", and tallying sugar grams. Skinny people see the food and eat it. They don't need a science lesson each time they want a muffin. Me neither, case closed.

I am sick and tired of portion control. I've got an entire collection of decrepit orange, older-than-dust, measuring cups in the kitchen drawer. Every time I open the drawer, they get jammed behind the cabinet causing me to shove, push, pull, and yank simply to figure out how many ounces of orange juice I get. The heck with that; I'm gulping down directly from the carton.

Don't even get me started on exercise! Dragging this drowsy old body out of bed and facing a half hour of wheezing and sweating up and down hills in a windy, cold, damp, dark, morning is not my idea of "healthy lifestyle. Turn off the alarm, snuggle up a little closer, and tell me it's Saturday. That's my idea of morning motivation.

Like I said, this "healthy lifestyle" thing is for the birds. It's not worth the effort anymore. Goodbye diet blues.

Oh sure, there's something to be said for the self-esteem and compliments from my friends. The back aches, fear of a heart attack, and darting down side corridors of the mall to avoid someone seeing how much weight I put on are also no longer a part of my itinerary. As for clothes getting too tight or buttons bulging on my shirt, that's in the rear view mirror too. And I do have to admit it is nice to be able to breathe after climbing a flight of stairs or to be able to touch my toes without a written plan...

Sigh...

OK, you win; I'll write one more week. But I am buying new measuring cups.

HEALTHY TRAVELS

Since the nature of a career of speaking to others about habit changes requires more than a fair amount of time "on the road," it behooves me to master the skill of eating healthy while travelling. Else wise, surviving on the "100% muffin, cookie, and pretzel diet" offered in planes and airports would cause me to gain back my weight — resulting in the loss of my livelihood and taking with it any credibility I might have in writing this column.

As I put pen to paper (more accurately "keyboard to word processor"), I find myself determined finally to be successful in my travel and dieting endeavors.

"Failure to plan," is "planning to fail." Therefore, utilizing all the marvels of the world wide web, I first researched which restaurants near my destination excel in "fit fare cuisine," and printed out maps with walking directions from my hotel to said establishments. By forsaking taxicabs, I am ensuring that I will get the requisite activity level to prevent weight gain.

Furthermore, should my body be a temple, than notice is hereby given that only the pure shall henceforth be allowed passage.

In my overstuffed carry-on suitcase, there is a food diary to record each calorie, taken directly from a booklet containing the nutritional makeup of more than 17,000 foods from five continents. Only those with the appropriate glycemic index shall be chosen.

To quench my thirst, I have opted for the clarifying, clear, cleansing choice of bottled water, rather than sucking down syrupy, sweet, sugary sodas. Instead of the unhealthful indulgence in a vodka martini to relax, I unwind with a delightful kiss of lime added to a refreshingly cold glass of tomato juice spiked with just a hint of Worchester sauce.

As for the omnipresent treats, nary an icing-covered, foil-wrapped, oatmeal cookie has yet crossed my lips. Moreover, those small, individually packaged trail mix bags with delectable chunks of lightly salted cashews, dried pineapple, and apricot bits, have gone untouched. Even the siren-like seductive summons of the tantalizingly crunchy, oh-so-delightful toffee-coated peanuts has fallen upon deaf ears.

I am convinced I've got this travelling thing mastered. Of course, the real test will come when I actually leave my driveway.

Veterans

Weary from an unending battle, we huddled as one, heads bowed, shoulders hunched, debating strategies. Moments before, we knew little of each other. Now, bonded by a common history and mission, we were uniting as brothers.

"How you holding out?" I asked of Jeff, the robust man to my left. I had not known him long, but my concern was authentic.

"It's tough. I thought I could do it, but lately —," his voice, thick with emotion, evaporated.

I grasped his shoulder. "I know. I've been there."

"We all have." Russ, the third of our triad, spoke, his words replete with compassion.

Jeff continued, "I was doing so well, down 44 pounds. I thought I had it together. Then, well, you know, we went on vacation. Since then, I've put back on 20. I can't get seem to get back in control."

"You'll get through this." I tried to be reassuring, hoping he wouldn't see my own unrelenting doubts. "It's a temporary setback; that's all, only a failure if you stop now."

Russ nodded as I spoke. "This is a lifestyle change; there will be good days and bad, ups and downs. The key is to keep on moving."

Russ pulled a snapshot of an extremely obese man by a pool from his pocket and placed it in front of us. The man in the photo seemed weighed down, not only by his immense mass, but also by a grey life-draining aura of fatigue that seemed to afflict the photograph itself.

"That was me," said Russ, "I lost 200 pounds." The gentleman across the table today had a thin frame, angular features, and abundant energy, belying his past. If not for a resemblance in his eyes, I would have passed off his statement as whimsical fantasy.

"Amazing," the word slipped from my lips involuntarily. I took a deep breath, renewed.

Russ smiled, radiating an understated, but well-deserved, pride of accomplishment.

"One day at a time," he said, "It's a struggle – but you get through it."

Jeff continued to study the photo. "Thank you both," he said. "I appreciate this."

It was time; we could delay no more.

"Ready?" I asked.

They nodded.

I turned to the waiter and waived away the chocolate cake, "We'll skip dessert."

The battle again was joined.

Noticing Joy

It is not possible to feel disheartened when in the presence of an infant's laughter.

Nothing so testifies to the glory and unlimited potential of all the universe's can be as much as the unrestrained, pure, spontaneous belly laugh of a delighted infant. Lacking judgment, shame, and fear, those heart felt giggles cascade unendingly from a baby's mouth, infectiously scattering awe, joy, and an affirmation of Life, giving voice to the jubilant song of the heart.

The first glow of a new romance makes all life fresh again. Elation bathes the soul, skin tingles electrically, and we become excited by each pump of our heart. In those early days, consciousness bursts forth with each morning sun, filling our view with a rich, detailed, and gloriously textured pastiche of our surroundings. What was blank is now a wide-ranging canvas of gleaming colors. Life flows through and around us, creating immunity from the careworn drudgeries of our daily reality.

I am made alive by the bracing scent of a desert autumn's first raindrops as they slip silently and softly through the dry, dusty, balmy sky. As the grime of all that was is cleansed from the atmosphere, and the first splattered drips bury themselves in the sand; I am at one with the essence of Mother Earth. Together, we are rinsed young again, the purifying fragrance infusing us with vigor to face unflinchingly the day.

These are glorious moments — frequently unnoticed.

In spite of that, they are just few of the easy joys of life, woven through the banal activities of daily grocery store excursions, checkbook balancing, and jury duty. Time and again, my existence devolves to a roll call of "to-dos" with no breathing space between items. I lurch zombie-like from waking to night, blinders attached, immune to these relaxed pleasures encircling me.

In those times, I mindlessly seek comfort, reaching for what works quickly, not well: a muffin, bag of chips, a handful of chocolate from my co-worker's desk.

Feed the heartbreak, starve the Soul.

Yet, if I pause for but an instant and look around, I can add to the glorious inventory of pleasures encompassing me each moment, and revel instead in the stronger, affirmative, sensation I receive from self-control, treating well my body, and letting fly my Spirit.

NEW LIFE AT 51

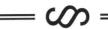

Darkness is banished; everything now radiates with the timeless magnificence of uncountable suns — and I am in touch with the grandeur of Life, feeling the newfound joy of an infant. All things are new again.

Be assured I have not stopped my meds. No Samaritan has approached me with fortunes from lost ancestors, and I have neither won the lottery, nor found an unexpected Picasso buried within Grandma's old trunk in the garage.

Today's gift is far more priceless.

For background, understand that I usually do consider myself to be an "adult." However, that does not mean I am pleased with the messy concept of mortality. I prefer — whenever possible — to retain the childlike view of the universe I had when protected from the fangs of that worldly reality by my parents (not then knowing they were probably doing the same as I do now).

Therefore, I have opted to not be "grown up," and resisted getting a routine colonoscopy, despite repeated reminders of its value. Beyond the "yick" factor I closely attached to such a procedure, the potential bursting of my bubble of immortality was too fear provoking. If one doesn't acknowledge what is frightful, it does not exist, right?

As I have adjusted diet and lifestyle to help alleviate the concerns of heart attack or stroke (most of the time), they do not elicit the gut wrenching horror in me that does cancer. Since my mother died savagely and before her time (or so I am convinced) from "the Big C," the slightest pain in my abdomen, or mole on my skin, whips up a frenzy of excruciating fear of following too soon in her path.

Simply look away; all unpleasantness will be gone. Resume breathing.

Alas, that lasts only so long. Being an "adult," I reluctantly consented to stagger fearfully into the dark place, my wife propping up my inner child. It's true, "the prep was worse than the process" (although the "prep" allows you to catch up on your reading).

Today, as I was handed the photographs of my colon, I beamed with the same pride as a new mother receiving her infant. Although I was told, "Nothing to worry about — see you in 10 years," what I heard was, "The future is yours again. Enjoy it."

I grew up a little today, yet I feel so much younger.

NIGHTLY REFLECTIONS

Each night while changing clothes, she purposely faced herself in the mirror — examining each curve, inspecting her shape, turning first left and then right, comparing profiles. It was as intertwined into her nightly routine as deeply as washing her face.

Four-plus decades under gravity's influence leave a discernible legacy. What was firm was now looser, what was thin was now thicker — and it seemed everything was in competition to see what could droop the furthest. Inside, she felt pretty much as she had since girlhood, yet outwardly, her body was being replaced by her mother's.

Of course, this nightly ritual of observation and analysis wasn't logical; after all, another transit of the earth could neither reduce inches nor relax the lines ever more obvious around her eyes. Nonetheless, the little girl inside never completely accepted that the years were here to stay. Maybe today would be different, just maybe…

On the bed, observing, sat her husband; he took that to be his responsibility in this nightly custom.

"You're watching me," she said without turning toward him, feeling his gaze.

"You're gorgeous," came the simple response.

"I don't know how you can say that," she replied, holding in her belly and monitoring her reflection. "I feel so fat."

"I think you get better looking every year. I can't wait until you're

80."

Turning from the mirror to face him, she saw that familiar, loving grin; his eyes still danced each time she met his gaze.

"I wish I saw myself the way you do," she said.

Rising from the bed, he joined her in front of the mirror. "Look at me: gray hair, crow's feet, more wrinkles than you — and these." He pinched the few extra inches of skin encircling his waist. "I could say the same thing. What do you see in me?"

"I love you," she replied. "You look great for 50. You make me laugh. You accept me for who I am."

"Back at you," he said.

In the mirror stood a middle-aged couple — all things considered, doing OK. Youthful days of tight, tan, firm bodies had receded; replaced with the wisdom of years, mutual respect from a good partner, and the friendship and love of a strong relationship. Measured by that light, they were stunning.

She took him by the hand, shut off the light, and left the mirror behind.

PRIORITIES

If Life is a journey, priorities form the road map.

Priorities are not all alike. For example, there are the trivial; "Honey, let's have potatoes instead of pasta." There are intermediate: "Do we refinance the house to pay for the kids' college?" And then there are enormous, powerful, life-changing ones to light our way and guide us to our final destination.

In philosophical discussions at dinner parties, the question arises, "In order, what are your three most important priorities?"

My well rehearsed reply rolls off my tongue, "Health, Family, Career." I know this because I am enlightened (and have engaged the service of fine therapists). Such topics matter to enlightened people.

I also accept that one might disagree (even I do at times); that misses the point. Rather, the issue here is "The Three" are so critical, I don't even have to think about it. Yet, therein lies a dichotomy: if they are so very important, why not reflect upon them more than I do?

I vocalize, "Health," then eat excessively, evade the doctor, and seek extensive rationale to avoid exercise. If health is my highest priority, I manifest it in an unusual fashion.

Second Priority: "Family." However, when my wife says, "let's play," resistance wells up; I just have so darn much work to do. She

— being the loving, supportive partner — gives me permission to enhance Priority Three: Career, and write my overdue speech. I opt instead to use those two hours adjusting the desktop photograph on my computer. After all, who can be productive when the scenery on screen is unattractive?

As a result of my inappropriate time management, Guilt makes its appearance — always a catalyst to eat blindly, medicate away my feelings, and insult my health. Voila, a cycle is complete!

If analyzed by what I do, rather than what I have memorized to impress people, would not my priorities be: "Eating, Procrastination, Guilt"? After all, that is what fills my days.

It's so easy to proclaim out loud what's essential (especially when directing others), yet it's not so effortless to actually follow through.

If health is truly my Priority One, I must act upon it.

I was going to conclude with sage advice on how you could adjust your priorities. But you'll excuse me if I instead put down this donut and take a walk.

THE CURSE OF PERFECTIONISM

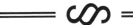

The alarm clock rattles, buzzes, and wretches. As I force myself to face my day, I am immediately overwhelmed with all I must complete, everything I must do — and immediately yank the blankets back over my head artfully, slamming the snooze button in one fluid motion.

There's always tomorrow; all things become possible in the new day. Today, I'll coast.

As a recovering perfectionist, I understand perfection is an impossible pursuit, yet for some unknowable reason I crave that title anyway. The hitch isn't my desire, it's my actions — or more accurately, lack thereof — caused by trying to be perfect instead of actually working to be better.

In past days, I thought I had to be "the perfect dieter:" avoiding EVERY snack, steering clear of ANY treats, and swearing off ALL nibbling. As life would have it, without thinking, I mindlessly munch a handful of nuts from my coworkers desk, a habit I've repeated countless times. Once I realize what I've just done, I am embarrassed and disappointed by my actions, as well as ashamed of my lack of willpower.

A decision is at hand. I mull my options, navigating the fierce storm raging within. I could consider this faux pas as human error, eat a little less tonight, congratulate myself for adjusting, and move closer to my goal.

Or, as a full member of Perfectionists United (known as "P.U."), chant our mantra (join me if you know the words), "As long as I blew it, I'll really blow it, and start again tomorrow." Soon therefore, an entire bowl of peanuts vanishes, as do extra brownies from the office party, and two bags of chips from the employee cabinet. I weigh more now than when the alarm blared.

What would have been a minor detour has become a full-stop road closure — because of my perfectionist objectives. When I try to break these bonds, they even slip cancer-like around my thoughts to undermine the cure: small consistent steps.

Fifty pounds is too much; five is not enough. Wait until you're ready to do it all. Running five miles is unrealistic; walking a block is useless. Sit down, relax; turn up the TV.

Black. White. Perfect. Awful. Success. Failure.

The world is nuanced with progress happening via minor movements; success gradually coalescing around the actions. One tentative step now, another thereafter — each a deliberate decision, each its own accomplishment.

I KNOW MANY THINGS

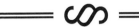

I have amassed great knowledge on many subjects.

I learned not to run with scissors while attending Botsford Elementary. At UCLA, I was infused with wisdom from the writings of Voltaire and Shakespeare. My time at the College of Hard Knocks has made me woefully aware that not everyone is as he appears.

I can recite the Gettysburg address, or at least the famous sections. My technological skills allow me to understand computers (and because I am snobby in such matters, I prefer Macintosh). I am admittedly unclear as to whether there are six or seven continents as I am unsure whether it's "Europe and Asia," or "Eurasia." Yet, I am knowledgeable enough to realize that on a grand scale, it matters little. Although, being worldly, I am aware that if I were a citizen of Europe and Asia, it would concern me more.

I can say "hello" in five languages — six Pig Latin is included.

I understand relationships, and how "one attracts more flies with sugar than with vinegar" (although I am unclear why I would wish to attract flies).

My curiosity about other beliefs is unbounded, as I know it is arrogance to assume that my beliefs are the "correct" ones. I have ascertained that those who claim "complete knowledge" obviously do not possess it.

I know to listen intently, not to interrupt, and never, ever, respond to the question, "Does this make my butt look big?" Experience is a cruel instructor.

Because I speak with enthusiasm, have gray hair, wear glasses, and can rub my goatee in a distinguished manner while pondering great thoughts, others seek my knowledge on topics of mind and body. Being wise, I recognize that "pondering" makes one seem more intelligent than "talking."

When questioned, "How do I lose weight?" I pontificate (post pondering), "Eat a little less than you want, walk a little more than you would, wait a moment longer than you think you can. Focus on today. Take small steps."

"Now we know!" they proclaim, overflowing with the joy of understanding and healing, lives now improved from my astute counsel.

Seeking knowledge — and knowing what to do with it — is actually quite simple, especially when instructing others. Putting it into practice on myself is something I still must learn.

A MAN AMONG WOMEN

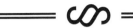

Although most men enjoy the company of the opposite sex, there are many who feel awkward in a room chock-full of women discussing weight loss, body image, and health concerns — a situation in which I find myself weekly. I enjoy the interchange. My wife says it puts me in touch with my "feminine side." Being sure of my masculinity, I understand that is a compliment and do not concern myself that it might diminish my manliness.

The barrel-bellied man new to the meeting did not seem so comfortable with his "feminine side" however. The only other male, he sat board-rigid, wordless, and stoic, a stubble of a beard dotting his heavy jowls. With an ocean of conversation swirling about, he remained motionless, holding his diet materials on his lap; his eyes fixed straight ahead, neither turning left nor right. Wearing working class, paint-stained, weather-beaten jeans hoisted over his large belly with thick suspenders, he contrasted starkly with the sea of bright colors, earrings, animated conversations — and estrogen.

He looked as at ease as a mouse at a convention of cats.

It was apparent he worked with his hands. I admire such men, as the period of boyhood where one learns to use tools and engines zipped by me. Being a bespectacled, obese child, I was ostracized and teased, and therefore spent my days alone with books — and food.

I reached out my hand to the stranger.

He returned the gesture, eager to talk to someone who didn't wear makeup. (I might have a feminine side but do draw the line at certain behaviors.) I expected his grip to be viselike; it was gentle.

"What brings you to the meeting today?" I pulled up a chair.

He appeared to size me up, determining if I could be trusted. Dropping my gaze and very intently studying the floor, he softly answered, "My wife's been on me for years to lose weight. I kept putting her off, told her I could do it on my own. But I kept gaining. I made excuses; she listened — until last night when she started crying and told me she's afraid I'm going to have a heart attack if I don't do something. She said that would kill her too; she loves me too much to watch that happen and I need to do something now."

He collected his thoughts. "She's my world. So, I'm here."

Sometimes we move forward on our own; other times we need a nudge. What matters is we're not alone.

THOSE WERE THE DAYS

I miss plopping myself on the sofa, watching TV late at night, a gallon tub of premium, chocolate fudge, brownie, mint swirl, marshmallow, cashew ice cream in my lap; decadently swirling the spoon along the edges of the carton (because that's the softer part and it doesn't bend the utensil).

Longingly, I remember buckets of extra-crispy, double doughy, steaming-hot, deep-fried chicken with moist mashed potatoes drowning under a pond of gravy; a soft, warm, flaky, slightly browned, oversized biscuit to soak it all up.

As a child, before days when LDL and triglycerides mattered, I looked forward to Sunday breakfast. Together we sat for a sugar-laden, high caloric, feast prepared lovingly by Mom. So much food filled the kitchen that it covered the table, a small tray, and overflowed on to the turquoise Formica kitchen counter.

Our ritual commenced with eggs scrambled with salami and cheese — real cheese, not the low fat imitation — in puddles of butter. Sharing the plate would be three pancakes, with syrup (and butter); onion rolls, bagels, cream cheese (or butter); and hash browns (fried in butter). In the event we finished the meal with even a thimble full of space remaining in our bellies, it was filled with seven-layer chocolate cake and black and white cookies. One never knows how long it'll be until the next meal; better eat up.

I long for those simple days.

Yet, I don't miss the embarrassment of pants so stretched that buttons popped off in history class, or so tight on my portly legs that the seam split while playing tetherball; sending me crying across the playground, mortified as the other children laughed at me.

As a teen, the girls in my neighborhood conducted a survey as to who was the best looking boy. Richard Gast came in first; my face came in second. I have no interest in returning to times when I was described as, "a great personality with a nice face."

"Great personality" was a euphemism I detested.

I have no desire to return to times of avoiding doctors, finding excuses not to meet new people, suffering chest pains, steering clear of family reunions, shopping in husky sections — and living merely to overindulge in ice cream, fried chicken, and big buttery breakfasts.

I do miss those childhood tastes upon my tongue; a day doesn't pass when I don't mourn my mother. However, I'm happier now than I was back then.

That's important to remember.

BACK TO NATURE

For me, exercise consists of walking to the grocery store to pick up a gallon of ice cream. I require goals; meandering wistfully along the beach — no matter how picturesque — doesn't fill that objective.

However, my wife insists we get "out in nature." I am unsure why this is essential. After all, I ride a bicycle and take a daily walk, both of which are outside the confines of my house. Isn't that "nature?"

I don't have a problem with "nature" per se; I'm just not sure where are its boundaries. How far from home must I go to be in it? Why isn't it closer? When I leave the window open, is not the breeze flowing through my screen, "nature"? Weekly, I brave the flora and fauna of my front law — all part of nature I presume — as I mow it. (My wife insists trimming the grass is as similar to "being in nature" as rearranging patio chairs is to landscaping.)

Don't get me wrong, I hold nothing against the great outdoors; I even watch the weather channel. It's just, that nature is so darn, well — how can I say this — "natural." I get cold in nature. Dirt gets on my clothing. When I go to Nature, I must put on special trail shoes with laces long enough to tie down an ocean liner. The extra loops and flaps on these shoes baffle me and make me feel stupid.

When my wife is bored, I inevitably hear, "Honey, let's do something different."

I hate that sentence; I know where it's going — and it's not inside.

"Such as?" I'll ask, hoping my preconceptions are wrong.

"I don't know. What would you like to do?"

See, this confuses me. I'm content doing what I'm doing or I would already be doing "something different." I enjoy doing things the same. I know how to do them.

"How about (… wait for it, wait for it…) we go to nature?"

I attempt to delay the fait accompli. "It's cold outside."

"Wear a jacket."

"It's windy."

"Put on a scarf."

"My scarf's itchy."

Accepting the inescapable, my cranky inner child bundles up in prickly neck wear, overstuffed coat, insulated gloves, and ski mask, to join my wife on the beach — perfectly timed for an arctic blast of freezing cold wind, carrying sharp pinpricks of icy sea mist to slam into my glasses, making it impossible to see.

Unaware of my trauma, she says, "Isn't this beautiful?"

Too wrapped in protection to move freely, I merely grunt, and imagine warmer times in my living room, staring out the window, observing nature where it belongs.

AFTER YEARS OF MARRIAGE

Boldly she wore pink; he, however, was timidly draped in brown. She exploded with brightness while the wood-grained walls of the airport restaurant swallowed him whole. She came forward; he fell back.

A gentle, refined seasoning of white complimented her look: sweater, sneakers, and beautifully coiffed hair. From my mother's day she came – and wore her age with proud, enthusiastic confidence.

His aura — sluggish and thick — was the perfect fit for his oversized waist and heavy movements. If not for her vibrancy to serve as a counterweight, he would have been invisible, absorbed by the background of the dimly lit restaurant.

Despite differences, their body language shared a history woven into long-term couples. They had seen much together; it was that bond that held them close.

He stared out the window, a leather-bound menu closed in front of him. Although the tarmac was busy, he was not watching the commotion; his eyes were fixed in space as he tried to remove himself from the discussion.

"What about your weight?" She asked. In her emphatic determination, there was no cruelty; simply the loving concern of a spouse who's had this same discussion time and again. Whereby it would be wise for others not to venture there, wives have privilege; they walk where most wisely do not tread. "I don't want to be a pest. It's just the doctor said if you don't watch what you eat, you'll have another heart attack."

"I'm tired of rabbit food," he said, struggling to hold down his emotion. "I want something real. When I'm done eating, I want to know I had a meal." He didn't look at her; he was speaking to the window.

"I know," she said, compassion in her voice. "Please..."

Interrupting the conversation, the waiter arrived.

Dropping her gaze at her husband, she turned to the waiter, "I'll have the chicken salad please. And a cup of tea."

He looked at her dark brown, dull gray partner, who didn't look up from the menu.

Waiting patiently, the waiter remained.

The husband broke the silence, quietly, softly, as he handed over the menu. "Chef's salad. Fat free dressing."

As the waiter left, the brown man turned back to the window, unable to see the pink and white glow of softness in his wife's eyes. Underneath the table, she patted his leg.

Together, silently, holding hands, they watched as airplanes took to the sky.

THE SALAD BAR

Today, dear traveler, we shall venture into the land of the salad bar, a glorious and wondrous place for dieters. Please keep hands and arms inside the bus as I assume the role of tour guide, enlightening you with tips for better consumption.

There are two types of bars: one consists of glass bowls of leafy lettuce, crinkle-cut carrots, and sliced celery, nested in clear cutlery that frustratingly swirl about in craters of ice, making it impossible to use the supplied (always incorrect) utensil to retrieve anything. Periodically, baby corn or garbanzo beans add some taste to this bland assortment of fibrous, flavorless, foods. Since such a salad bar is indeed simply a "salad bar," there is no reason to maximize intake. Just grab a small plate and be done. After all (I don't mean to be cynical), who cares?

However, the hosts of heaven sing when we spy a long-row, deluxe, salad bar, whereby tomatoes and mushrooms are present merely to give the title "salad bar" a smidgen of authenticity. Upon moving down the aisle, twisting and bending to avoid the annoying "sneeze shield" (which is never correctly placed) we venture into exciting terrain, commencing with olives (green and black), pickles, pasta salad, macaroni salad, potato salad, and carrot salad. This hodgepodge of sub salads is reason enough to rejoice; yet the rumbling joy in one's belly is merely beginning.

We leave the concept of "salad" in our wake as we can load our plate with thick fried potatoes, tater rounds, French fries, and mashed potatoes. A multicultural experience commences as fried chicken, mini-tacos, pizza, and egg rolls share space with sushi, tempura, and spaghetti; leaving just enough room for a bowl of cheddar cheese, cream of potato, or taco soup.

While steadying precariously this collected cornucopia of caloric courses, add crackers (saltine or breadstick), bread, rolls, and a bagel; each slathered with butter, cream cheese, or peanut butter. Hang from the thumb, the wire tray compilation of aluminum tins holding a treasure trove of flavored jams, jellies, and preserves.

With experience, one can further learn to balance chocolate, vanilla — or the more exotic tapioca pudding. A second bowl allows for a choice of three flavors of ice cream, chocolate syrup, maraschino cherries, and of course whipped cream.

One might wonder why I have strayed from discussing salad dressings (next to the impulse items: bacon bits, croutons, sunflower seeds, raisins, peanuts, and crispy fried noodles). It would be wrong; after all, one chooses salad bars to watch one's weight.

THE RULES

We are raised to follow rules.

The process begins as children with "small rules," whereby penalty for infraction is a "time out," a mind-numbingly dull exile to bedroom isolation, where all I could do was stare at a faded yellow wall as the clock ticked away hours. Over time, I came to understand the cost of such banishment was not worth breaking house regulations. Therefore, I came home by curfew, attended school when I'd rather be at the beach, and dutifully dragged the bent, steel garbage can to the curb each Tuesday night. Following rules gave me freedom.

"Big rules" are called "laws," where violations result in extreme unpleasantness enforced by well-trained strong men with crisply ironed blue uniforms and black steel weapons at their sides. Those who break these rules sacrifice self-determination through long-term adult "time outs" behind metal bars.

Being somewhat compliant, I operate within the confines of rules. I pay taxes by April 15, do not drive 80 miles an hour, and attempt to treat others the way I want to be treated. Because of adherence to these edicts, my life usually flows more smoothly.

So, here's the thing: Despite the fact that I obey the law; honor codes of ethics, and follow behavioral etiquette, I remain perplexed by my periodic futile attempts to ignore the most powerful, omnipotent, and all-pervasive "Prime Rule of the Universe" which is, "the Universe will not change its rules to accommodate my whims, fantasies, and desires." Simply put, "If I always do what I've always done, I'll always be where I've always been." Ignorance is no excuse; there is no court of appeals, clemency does not exist.

Yet I proclaim, "This time will be different; I'll lose the weight. This time, I'll be perfect." Although — aside from more enthusiastic lip service — I don't actually DO anything differently from all the OTHER times I espoused that same pronouncement. Soon, frustrated and angry again, I grumble about my results (or lack thereof), as they are exactly what they were each previous time I did the same thing. "Why?" I ask. "This isn't fair!"

Undeterred by reality, I persist, repeatedly hurling myself into the same patterns, expecting new results. Finally, exhausted and defeated, I realize that instead of walking into walls, I can open a door. I obey the rules and try a new approach; I change.

"IT" will never be different. "I" must be different. Those are the rules. And once I accept that, I set myself free.

WHAT CHOICES PUT HIM THERE?

It was a most unlikely sight.

He — late thirties, looking older — supported a worn, faded, red backpack over his denim jacket as he trudged down our street. What drew my attention however was the bright yellow blanket with large blue stars and comets draped over his right shoulder; obviously a child's. The apparent reason for this colorful cloth was the small boy holding his father's hand as they headed down the street.

Earlier, on my morning walk, our paths crossed a few miles from here. At that time, he carried the sleeping boy over his shoulder, wrapped in the cosmically decorated fabric. It is curious to witness a man transporting a small blanket-wrapped youngster through the morning streets, so I offered assistance.

"Nah," was his reply. "I just need a ride. But thanks."

He continued walking; hoisting the child, while his free hand — with thumb outstretched — sought to hitch a ride.

Since then, an hour had passed and the boy was walking — tiredly — with his father carrying the blanket. Each time a car whizzed by, dad extended his thumb. Each time, the driver paid no heed and the duo trudged on. Together, one unit, repeating the pattern, they continued down the sidewalk and I watched them shrink and disappear into the distance.

The uniqueness of their plight caused me wonder. What choices had he made to put them here today? Were they poor decisions and now he was paying a price? If he had known the future, would he have acted differently? What circumstances put a father and son together, walking miles, seeking transportation, adorned in a bright yellow blanket on a cloudy, misty morning? It is so surprising the decisions others make. Why don't they think it out? Don't they see?

I entered my house to change my clothes and faced the mirror. Five decades leaves its calling card: what was firm is soft, what was flat now sags. Was this my doing? It is simple to dissect others' actions, complacently directing their lives. But when the reflection looking back is one's own, smugness quickly evaporates.

What choices had I made to put me here today? Was I now paying a price? If I had known my future, would I have acted differently? Did I think it out? Didn't I see?

He did what he did, and is where he is — as am I. Resentment, judgment, and regret serve no purpose. Yet tomorrow remains wide open with all things possible. Decisions do matter; I must choose wisely.

GOTTA GET OUT MORE

There are countless words describing my childhood; "athletic" is not one.

But when the merry tinkling of the ice cream truck drifted across hot summer afternoons on Rensellor Avenue, I would sprint and leap like a gold medalist on springs. Catching sight of my 150 pound, four-foot-tall frame barreling down the sidewalk, quarter in hand, hellbent for chocolate coated ice cream was a jaw-dropping spectacle. If I stretched out my arms, I would have achieved liftoff.

Over time, I learned to temper my outward exuberance for treats, figuring if no one saw me eat, they wouldn't notice I was fat. Mind you, I didn't actually stop eating loads of sugar; I just didn't barrel full-steam down the street to get them like some out-of-control locomotive. Instead I opted for more discreet methods such as shaving small slivers from cake instead of taking a slice (making it less apparent to the untrained eye that I had eaten some), or hiding chocolate in my clothes (always a special treat for mom on laundry day — especially if she didn't inspect my pockets first).

If a tree falls in the woods, yes, it does make a sound. So too, if a pound cake is consumed stealthily, it retains its calories. Concealing food does nothing to disguise the results; a 44 inch waist being a reliable indicator of surplus caloric consumption — even if no one observes it.

Please forgive my youthful transgressions, as I was then addled from a non ending influence of high fructose corn syrup and have come to see the error of my ways, opting now for skim milk (called "the blue stuff" by professional dieters), high fiber breads ("cardboard") and fat free cheeses ("rubber").

Fast forward: My wife went to visit family this week, leaving me to fend for myself. No one will mistake me for a chef, but I do OK. Insert in microwave. Hit start. Peel cardboard. Consume. I won't write any cookbooks; but I don't starve either.

Being lonely, I wanted a "fun food;" you know, something special, a rare treat. Yet years of discipline have left their toll and I begrudgingly opted for salad.

While resigning myself to the doldrums of leafy greenery, I noticed a bottle of full-calorie, creamy white, ranch dressing — the real stuff, not that gelatinous fat-free goop mislabeling itself as "tasty."

With bold abandon, I measured one full tablespoon and poured it right on top of my salad; plain as day. In full view — and I didn't care! What a thrill seeker am I! And then, I ate it — in daylight — just like that!

At that moment I realized I really have to get out more.

Chubby children and strict parents

When people ask what I do for a living, I reply that I speak on "increasing happiness, improving productivity, and enhancing the quality of life for recovering perfectionists." Many relate; some even hire me. Because of this background, I was intrigued by a study from the Boston University School of Medicine that appeared in the June issue of *Pediatrics*, which pointed out that strict mothers were nearly five times more likely to raise overweight first-graders than mothers who treated their children with flexibility and respect while also setting clear rules. Other observations dotted the study but that one point lit brightly for me.

I propose a theory as to why strict parents might tend to raise chubby offspring.

If I (speaking as an adult) believe I'm "good" or "bad;" "right" or "wrong;" "perfect" or "awful;" with no "inbetweens," then all transgressions are equally wrong and all errors are equally harmful once I cross "the line." In other words, as long as I'm "off" my diet, there is no difference between being "off," "Off," or "OFF!" It's equally dark anywhere in "Off land," and since I'm not ready to return to the light and will face the same consequences no matter what I do, I might as well "get it all out of my system" so that when I return to the "right" side, I'll be free of the siren call of indulgence. That thought, of course, intensifies the damage caused by slip-up.

If however, I understand most behaviors are not "black and white," I realize there is a gradient in their results; I adjust sooner, incur less damage, and might actually feel proud of those adjustments.

Although I am able to explain that concept in about 100 words, taking it to heart — even in my fifties — is not so easy. I know it, sure. I even believe it. Yet, when I'm knee deep in the big muddy, it's hard to remember to I can turn around now.

Children have less reasoning ability than do adults (with some noted exceptions). They see black and white, good and bad, right and wrong; a clear line once crossed that has no nuances. Zero-tolerance guidelines might help when the child is in compliance, but once violated, one cookie is the same as the bag.

The key is kindness, support, guidance, and understanding; excellent advice for children—even those of us with gray hair and wrinkles.

THE BEST DAY OF MY LIFE

The summer of my 18th year was the first time I was thin. Attending college, The Moody Blues, Led Zeppelin, and the Rolling Stones blasted from my AM car radio. I walked precincts for my first election, wrote poetry in the evening, and was within daily driving distance from warm beaches (fueled by 30 cent-a-gallon gasoline).

The passing of seven years found me as a Northern California DJ spinning 45s from Van Halen, Joe Jackson and the Rolling Stones. I spent evenings in Community Theater, weekends producing a newsletter, and drove to work each morning, many times from different apartments. Life was sensuous, seductive, and skyrocketing.

As the calendar flipped through my thirties, I managed radio stations, bought a house, and began to feel I was making a difference in my community. I attended media conventions, interviewed celebrities, and covered the walls with collectible memorabilia from REO Speedwagon, Tears for Fears, and (you guessed it) The Rolling Stones. At day's end, a smiling, toothless, applesauce-covered face with deep blue, innocent eyes and wildly enthusiastically kicking feet in a high chair buoyed my spirits. Could life be better?

Sometimes, I think of the past with an almost sacred reverence. Those years prior to present day troubles were a richly colored, beautifully woven, warmly textured patchwork of memories. Conflict was nonexistent; mortality was unknown, and family celebrations always took place under sunny skies.

I long to return.

Or do I?

Despite the electricity of my teenage years, I felt powerlessness all too often, angry at the direction of my parents' generation. Though my twenties, bill collectors were common, furniture was made of cardboard, and my automobile starting in the morning was cause for celebration. The next decade ended with the scale reading 250 pounds, my marriage in divorce, and the health problems of each.

Lamenting the passing of what no longer exists — and never actually did — holds me captive. To fully appreciate Today (which is all the time I truly have), it's essential I stop frittering my time watching the rearview mirror and ignoring the beauty in front of me. Every moment is precious, vibrant, and brilliant, even while marked with blemishes and imperfections.

Today, I feel respected, healthy, and loved. I can squander these moments or inhale deeply that pleasure and savor the moment.

Today is the best day of my life; I can't wait to see tomorrow.

THINK ABOUT IT

"What are you thinking about?"

"Huh?"

"You look so deep in thought. I was just wondering what you're thinking about."

"Oh, um, well… nothing really. Just thinking."

"How can you think about 'nothing?' Do you imagine 'everything' covered by a big red circle with a diagonal slash over it?"

"Don't be cute. You know I hate that. Since you need to know more, I was just thinking about 'stuff.' Is that better?"

"'Stuff.' Hmmm. That covers a wide range. Is it philosophical 'stuff' like the sound of one hand clapping? Is it practical 'stuff?' Paying the bills, cleaning the house? Or do you allow your 'stuff' to fly on flights of fancy and think of tropical islands with open-air huts and warm breezes? 'Stuff' encompasses a lot you know."

"Jeeze, you're nosy. If you must know I was thinking about food."

"Ahh. Now we're getting somewhere. Can you be more specific? You seem to drift toward the vague."

"Sorry, I didn't know I had to run everything by you to make sure the details were hashed out."

"Hashed out? Food again?"

"Fifty thousand comedians are out of work and you're cracking wise! No, that comment was not food related."

"Sounds like we're making progress. So tell me about food. Do you think about food all the time?"

"No, just when I'm awake. When I'm sleeping, I dream about it."

"Now who's being cute?"

"OK, but they're my thoughts, not yours. I can be cute with them if I want to. Seriously, when I'm eating breakfast, I'm thinking about what to have for lunch. At lunch, it's dinner. After dinner, I think about eating anything that's slow enough to stick a fork into it."

"Sleeping cats better be nervous, huh?"

"It's not funny. Food sometimes feels like an obsession. It's hard to stay on my diet when I'm always thinking about what to eat."

"I was wondering —"

"Oh, I hate it when you start sentences like that. You're really trying to put another thought in my head and you think I won't notice it if you start with 'I was wondering.'"

"As I said, I was wondering… How would it feel if instead of saying 'Dieting is hard,' you said, 'Eating healthy is exciting. I feel great when I do it.' That's true too, isn't it?"

"Well, yeah. I just don't know if I can."

"Tell you what. Put me in touch with the guy who controls your thoughts and we'll fix you up and get back to you."

"Ouch."

"Yeah, I can be snarky sometimes. But if you change the way you look at it, you might do better, wouldn't you agree?"

"It's worth a thought."

Things that go
yum in the night

My sons finished their pizza and departed for the evening's events. My wife was asleep upstairs, leaving me unaccompanied in the silence of the night. Not a sound was to be heard, save the creaking of settling hardwood floors and the whispering lingering melody of wind chimes on the darkened front porch.

From the kitchen, hauntingly and gently, I hear, "Scott."

Startled, as I thought I was alone, I seek out the source of the voice. The door to the stairs remained silently and tightly closed. Both boys were still gone, and I was convinced neither of our cats could articulate my name so distinctly.

Again: "Hey, Scott. In here."

There was no mistake. Uneasily, I entered the kitchen, trying to hold down the cold, creeping, convulsions climbing my spinal column.

This is where it gets weird.

As I live and breathe, the leftover pizza on the table was calling to me in an eerie, enticing, siren-like, hauntingly seductive intone.

A brief digression is in order. If you've never had to battle a weight problem, right about now, you're probably putting down the newspaper, shaking your head in disgust, thinking I've had one too many slices of Hawaiian, deep-dish, heavy-on-the-mushrooms, extra saucy triangles of pizza and am writing while encased in a mind-altered pepperoni hallucination. Yet, those who struggle with each calorie are — at this exact same moment — nodding their heads enthusiastically in agreement, tapping this print, shoving it under somebody's nose, proclaiming victoriously, "See, I told you! Pizza does call out to me!"

What makes this so especially sinister is that the food waits until no one else is around to hear its call. Seeking to lure us into a vise-like grip, in the wee hours it chants, "Just one piece won't hurt," or "Come on, you know you want it."

Not only is pizza garrulous, its knowledge of psychology is worthy of a treatise. I, as a 51-year-old, can resist the urge to steal, cheat, and lie; yet find myself a powerless infant to the calling of the One Most Cheesy.

Knowing my weakness, I muster all my power and thrust the loquacious doughy demon down the disposal and flip the switch, victorious this time over its taunts.

BEING MEAN

Before I venture down this road, it is prudent of me to inform you of my past.

Ten pounds at birth, and always overweight as a child, my mother was troubled because other babies pushed away the bottle when full; I never did. I also recall unmistakably the humiliation of being the fattest child on the playground and the mortification of showering in front of other boys after gym class. Even at adulthood, the low self-esteem that marked my youth required years of therapy to wash away.

Understand please I don't wish those experiences on any child; as I move forward.

According to the AP, there is debate about how to label the condition of heavy children. Currently they are said to be "at risk for overweight" if their body-mass index (BMI) is between the 85th and 94th percentiles; in other words, they weigh more than 85 to 94 percent of their peers (based on historical averages). They're called "overweight" if their BMI is the 95th percentile or higher. The American Medical Association, and others, are considering changing this and using the same terms applied to adults — "overweight" or "obese."

Labeling a child obese might "run the risk of making them (or their family) angry," but it addresses a serious issue head-on, said Dr. Reginald Washington, of the American Academy of Pediatrics obesity task force. "There are a thousand reasons why (obesity) is out of control … one of them is no one wants to talk about it."

Obese "sounds mean. It doesn't sound good," said Trisha Leu, 17, who thinks changing the terms is wrong.

Following is what I believe.

Having been "there," "mean" was being taunted mercilessly as a teenager for having so much extra weight that it appeared I had breasts.

"Mean" was being the last one chosen to play kickball and listening to my teammates curse their rotten luck.

"Mean" was overhearing girls in high school describe in explicit detail how dreadful it would be to kiss me.

"Mean" was binge eating to erase the day's pain, only to have it return worse with morning's light.

I have compassion — and concern — for our children; one can feel both simultaneously. From my experience however, it is far "meaner" to mask reality with insincere descriptions, condemning them to unhealthy futures, than it is to educate honesty, informing them that although their weight does not determine self-worth, it does affect wellbeing. Then, we guide them gently to a healthier lifestyle with support and love. How about we even accompany them on their path?

That would be the nice thing to do.

THEORETICAL VERSUS ACTUAL

Today *(as planned):*

- Arise early smiling and refreshed; greet world with 45-minute brisk walk while listening to singing birds under sunny blue skies. Stop at coffee shop and read the paper; joyously greeting each person. Eat a healthy, balanced, nutritious breakfast while connecting with my wife. Drink three glasses of filtered water as a treat.

- Answer all e-mail. Write my column; infused with wit and insight. Send materials to three potential speaking opportunities, confident they'll hire me for twice asking price. Complete assignments for all clients prior to promised deadlines.

- Reconcile credit card statements, set up automatic banking to pay each and every bill for next three years. Buy groceries. Straighten office.

- Have lunch with a friend. Sit in the sun on a swing, singing. Watch entertaining, uplifting video. Have a wine cooler. Relax. Count blessings.

Today *(actual):*

- Got up late after throwing alarm with annoying buzzer at wall. Dragged my panting, sweaty, dreary, flabby body around the block for 10 minutes. Gagged down chalky instant breakfast while watching exercise infomercial. Waved to wife as she went to work. Decided extra caffeinated coffee is a "need," not a "want."

- Spent 45 minutes sifting through email about sexual potency, mortgages, and African expatriates offering me money. Stared at blank page while occasionally pounding head on desk to alleviate writer's block. (Took several aspirin.) Made one phone call where I was relegated to "voice mail hell" for 24 minutes. Cursed at automated voice. Slammed down phone; breaking mouthpiece.

- Shoved bills from one messy pile to another. Decided to scrape green fuzz off last week's leftovers for dinner. Came to terms with the fact that my office will always look like it was designed by tornado.

- Had three-hour chocolate binge fest; felt guilty (and fat) so I blamed my wife for having snacks in the house. (Learned new definition to "unwise decision.") Weather was cloudy so I zoned out with two martinis in front of TV while watching imbecilic sitcoms (which, in my mood, actually seemed appealing). Fell into restless sleep on couch, with face in drool stain on pillow.

Someone said happy simply accept life on its own terms. As my Yiddish grandmother Zlate said (in addition to countless repetitions of "Oy Vay"), "Mann plant Gott lach;" translated, "Man plans, God laughs." I must remember it's not about getting it done. It's about how I feel about what was done. It's not how far I have to travel, it's how far I have come.

Today: not so good. I was frustrated. But tomorrow, I try again. That's excellent.

REAL FOOD FOR REAL MEN

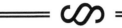

A man's gotta do what a man's gotta do.

And right now, after months of lightweight food with no taste — and even less heft — I've got a heavy hankerin' for a triple-meatball, pepperoni sausage, six-cheese submarine sandwich, oozing over a warm, doughy foot long toasted Mozzarella Parmesan Italian roll, followed by a family-size order of cottage fries (sans family) smothered in chili cheese sauce. The chaser for this gloriously caloric feast will be a chocolate chunk, hyper-sized, milk shake stuffed with peanut butter blobs and overflowing with rich syrup.

I'm a-fixin' to eat me something solid — and once I've got it in my mind, my diet is history.

I suck in my gut, march boldly into the sandwich shop, and swagger to the counter. Feet resolutely planted, I stand my ground in an oh-so-macho fashion and make direct eye contact with the young woman behind the register. Actually, I don't know if young women consider middle-aged, slightly soft, bespectacled, grey-haired men to be manly, but red meat, elevated-cholesterol, saturated-fat meals seem to me a masculine food; I must place myself in the right frame of mind prior to ordering.

She asks, "What would you like?" (I am amazed she is not swooning from the animal magnetism I exude.)

"Forget the calories, Scott; go for it!" I hear in my head.

Clearing my throat, I deepen my voice, and — for causes unbeknownst to me — reply in a crackling, tinny, scratchy sound, "Veggie sandwich. Diet soda."

Sean Connery had entered the restaurant; Woody Allen had ordered.

In my mind, I'm pounding my forehead with the heel of my hand, screaming, "What in Heaven's name are you doing? You passing up the mother lode of meats for sprouts and cucumbers again! Have you no pride?"

Over my internal din, I hear her ask, "Anything else?"

Ah-ha, an opportunity to redeem myself! Go for it Scott! Take the plunge; live on the edge! There's still time.

"No mayo please — and light on the cheese."

Arggh! It's as if I'm channeling elderly English ladies at high tea. Next thing you know, I'm going to tastefully chew ladyfingers while eating with my pinky in the air.

I see myself a ferocious carnivorous lion, chasing prey across the African savannah; yet, what repeatedly materializes is my inner bunny, nibbling carrot tops at the petting zoo.

Other people eat red meat without stress. What's wrong with Me?

The blood pounds loudly in my temples. "Wait!" I blurt out, "I want to change my order."

"Yes?" She looks up, knife poised to cut the bread.

"Give me extra spicy mustard. I can handle it."

End of the rat race

In younger days, everything was equally urgent and all things were critical. Was she adorned in the latest fashions? Did he have the hottest car? Were they vacationing at the fanciest locales? Missing one step would devastate an entire month's image.

Something unreachable, invisible, just out of grasp, was always required to complete their happiness, leaving an unfilled void at all times. Someday, they might find "It" and then, suddenly, like the sun breaking through a stormy sky, everything would be perfect. Until then, additions kept coming, agendas overflowed, and dollars kept draining. Constantly striving for perfection, most times they overlooked what was good.

Their schedule was no longer their own. Fighting traffic for hours in late model autos serving as communication central, entertainment centers, and even mobile kitchens, they would text message "I love you" to each other a few times a day so they would have at least have some connection. Over time, even that became a pre-programmed memo stored in speed dial — intimacy with an efficient edge.

As the future became the past, the bills mounted, the pressures piled — the treadmill snapped.

"I'm not happy anymore," he said. He wasn't looking at her; instead his eyes were fixed on the almost-consumed cake with "Happy

45th" on the top. The guests had departed and his words bounced off blank walls and echoed as they fell heavy to the floor between them.

She was neither angry nor surprised. He was merely the first to say out loud what they both felt.

Marriage counseling, frustration, and crying (by both of them): a long road back but they made it. They had tried so hard to do everything perfectly, to lead a fantasy life; it almost cost them their own.

Now — tonight — she watched him cut through "75 Years Young" on the white frosting as the crowd sang "Happy Birthday," no one more enthusiastically than she.

When the guests left, as they lay in bed, he reached out and squeezed her hand gently.

"I love you more than I knew I could," he said as he was drifting off to sleep, "You're as beautiful as ever. I'm so lucky."

His eyes closed, a smile fixed on his lips.

Staring into the mirror across the bed, she saw deep lines etched in her face, white in her hair, spots on her skin, and a lovely, sleeping elderly man beside her. She put the book in her lap down, shut off the light, slipped under the blankets behind him, putting her head on his back and as she closed her eyes.

Funny how things turn out, everything now was as close to perfect as she ever imagined.

MY CONFESSION

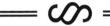

Since my age was counted in single digits, I've been dieting. If I assembled in one place all the pounds I've lost (and found again), it would sink a whale. I scan food packaging for terms like "low fat," "sugar free," or "no calories." I record how many glasses of water I drink and how many miles I walk. I weigh myself week in and week out in special pre-weighed "weigh in clothes." (I even know my belt weights 3.4 ounces, how's that for detail?) I speak to audiences around the country on the topic and, of course, I write this column, which is printed in several cities.

Everyone who knows me — and I mean EVERYONE — understands I am a professional dieter. There must therefore be at least a glimmer of recognition inherent in that knowledge that I just might have a few "issues" about eating.

So why do I try to keep it secret when I slip up on my program? It's as if by not admitting my error, no one will notice my weight problem. Granted, since I'm currently at my (mostly) correct weight, some might be shocked at what I can pack away in a binge. But — can I be honest? When I sported a 44-inch waist and topped 250 pounds — someone, somewhere, might have had an itsy-bitsy inkling that I could be squirreling away a few tortilla chips now and then.

Yet, I ate in secret. I hid food in my bedroom (and car... and closet... and dresser... and — well, you get the image). If the last slice of cake was missing — and no one else was around — I'd still shake my chocolate smudged face boldface denying 'twas I who finished it.

"Gremlins must have eaten it," my mother would say.

I'd nod my head as if chubby, unworldly beings really did sneak into the kitchen and make off with the baked goods. She said nothing else. I remained silent.

Here's the thing. Even now, admitting I overeat makes me ashamed of my weakness. My critical parent screams at my compliant kid (therapists will love that sentence), "You're a failure! What's wrong with you?"

So I deny the deed. The result? Guilt for being dishonest replaces the shame.

Either option inspires more eating to medicate the pain. If guilt and shame were motivational, I'd be bone skinny.

My way out is to own my problem, boldly and upfront. Therefore, at the risk of bursting your bubble, I stand before you to announce I slip up. I make mistakes. I err. I'll probably do it again. Hard to believe I'm not perfect, huh?

Please understand that. I'll do the same for you.

Stop that right now!

What are you looking around for? You know I'm talking to you. Yes, you — no, not the guy behind you. I'm speaking to YOU. Look at me; quit pretending you think I'm referring to someone else.

Now, just stop; it's for your own good. We both know it.

Yes, I know you're busy. You have so many responsibilities and commitments. But that's not going to fly this time. We're all busy. We're all overloaded. It's a matter of priorities, plain and simple. This time, make it work, OK?

Oh, more excuses? Well, welcome to Excuse Central pal; know 'em all. Got 'em all right here. "Just a little bit won't hurt." "I deserve it; it's been a tough week." How about this one: "When things settle down, I'll do it." I don't mean to be rude or crude, but the only time things will totally settle down is when six friends are carrying you away in a box.

Of course, there's always my favorite: "I can stop whenever I want." Yeah, right. If you can stop anytime, why did you let it get so out of control?

Do you enjoy unending aches and pains? Isn't it just oodles of amusement avoiding the dark side of the closet because you're afraid those unused clothes "shrunk" since you last wore them? Are we having fun now?

And finally, the ultimate kick in the pants: that undisguised glance in someone's eyes when she can't cloak how surprised she is by how large you've become since she last saw you. Just makes you feel warm all over doesn't it? Sure, sure, she covers it quickly; after all, she's not trying to be rude. But for that moment — that one, brief, instantaneous, short-lived, horrifyingly candid, flash — your sole desire is to drop through a hole in the floor. Honestly, do you really want to deal with that again? How many times will you avoid friends to prevent that from happening?

What's that? You DON'T like those feelings? Oh, good, we're making progress. But you don't have the energy to change?

I hear you! But, how much energy does it take for the 24-hour discomfort in your own skin? Or missing out on your kid's lives because you're too tired to play? How much of your precious lifeforce do you waste feeling bad about yourself every thinking moment of each and every day? Makes the effort more worthwhile, doesn't it?

Ready to stop now? Good. I'm pleased for you.

Step one is stop talking to this mirror; get out there, and take a walk.

KEEP A GOOD THOUGHT

My wife and I tried breaking our nightly routine. To alleviate muscle aches, we deduced that if we each slept on side of the bed where the other person usually lies, we might arise pain free. (It made sense in the moment.)

I make no claim that swapping pillows is a valiant act of bravado. That does nothing to diminish the reality that it, in fact, was awkward. Not simply "I-normally-don't-wear-this-color-so-I-feel-like-everyone's-staring-at-me" unpleasant; it was more akin to "Did-I-forgot-to-zip-something?" anxiety. We tossed, turned, bumped into each other multiple times, and waited twitchily for the arrival of Hypnos, the God of Slumber, only to be jilted on the mattress. After several fidgety hours, reverting to positions of yore, we obtained at last a modicum of shuteye.

It's not as if my bride and I, while writing our vows, discussed who would lay claim to which side of the bed. "Do you, Scott, promise to love, cherish, and support Mary Ann until the end of your days — while swearing to snooze faithfully on the section of bed furthest from the nightstand?"

No, that's not how it happens. Customs emerge. One moment, it's an arbitrary behavior, next instant: Habit. Isn't that how it is?

We set up repetitive behaviors for our ease; then, something alters them. We are naked, abandoned, and lonely. Without habit's landmarks, direction is lost; uneasiness swamps us. So, we rush back as quickly as possible, reassured finally by the embrace of the familiar.

This morning, as I left our home, I mentioned to my wife, "Keep a good thought." Neither a particularly sage nor unique turn of phrase, its sentiment is kind, and I meant it sincerely. Yet, it's another of those expressions that rolls off the tongue without thought: another habit.

And as I routinely walked 17 minutes down E Street and 11 minutes back on F Street (stopping at the regular time at "my" coffee house so I could sit at "my" table with a daily cup of coffee and read the morning newspaper), I realized how much of life is ordered on preset molds.

Awakening and sleeping are based on the clock. Workday functions are a matter of rote. Even my attitude is usually balanced. When events go awry — just as habitually — I eat to handle stress, then walk to handle the eating. Habits, patterns, routines everywhere.

I'm not complaining (mostly). I am fortunate; my challenges are less than those faced by many others. But that does not preclude me from wondering what I would see if I more often "shook it up" and did something off my beaten path, experiencing life with atypical eyes?

A good thought; one I must remember.

BEFORE I BEGIN...

I earn my living speaking. I feel alive when delivering motivational, energetic presentations to enthused audiences. Yet the irony is I spend most of my time isolated, without employees, working from an office in my house while my family is gone. Hour after hour slides by as I tap relentlessly on keyboard, stare at computer monitor, and write — alone.

Leading a solitary life, I have learned to be somewhat organized; I have no staff to assist me. Granted, I periodically curse and rant when I cannot find that which I seek because of poor filing. Gratefully, I am not on the other end of the spectrum bellowing, "Where are my glasses?" only to have my wife call back, "You're wearing them."

As I said, I keep things in their place — mostly.

That does not forgo within me an interest in improving my organizational skills. Therefore I made an appointment with a professional organizer. These dedicated denizens of domestic direction and design are on the front lines in the battle against entropy; expanding our horizons with hanging files, work zones, and paper flow. The results, I'm informed, are increased productivity, less stress, and a "reclaiming of one's space." This I find to be a highly respectable goal because credit card receipts, unsolicited faxes, and projects I'll do "one of these days" too often claim my space and battle to take it back. (As an aside, I found assurance — and humor — in the fact that the Professional Organizer lost my address.)

Yet, I digress.

Before her arrival, I found myself busily straightening my work-space, shredding papers, dusting shelves, and lugging boxes. Somewhere between chronologically ordering my CD collection, and using a ruler to make sure all wall hangings were parallel and equally spaced, the folly of my operation struck me.

I need her help but act as if I don't. I did not want her to realize my flaws. Gasp! She'll think I'm human!

It brought me back to promising I would return to my weight loss meetings AFTER I lost "those five pounds." Huh? How'd that work the last 16 times I did that? Do I truly believe people can't tell I'm having trouble on my diet unless I seek help? I hefted a 44-inch belly, and convinced myself that holding in my stomach would fool others to believe I had six-pack abs. Amazing how we can fool ourselves, isn't it?

Even powerful people have needs. Admit it. Embrace it. Correct it. It's actually surprisingly empowering to "own" who you are.

Oops, gotta go. I just noticed the maid is coming and I have to clean the house before she arrives.

AMAZING!

$$\infty$$

As they ambled up the slope to the restaurant, it was apparent the toddler was new to the concept of walking unaided, holding her mother's hand for security. From behind, her small body was obscured by a lavender backpack that bounced, as if bobbing on waves, with every step. This carryall obscured her frame from heels to head, and was adorned with a joyful smiling purple pony. Above the daypack was a forest of thick, dark brown hair, fashioned into a spout. Below were matching purple pony sneakers that lit up with each footfall.

The path before her held no interest. I — on the other hand — following behind was deserving of intense scrutiny. Her backward glances, coupled with forward movement, and yet-untuned walking skills came together. The result was she tripped and tumbled forward, catching herself before her small face made contact with the floor.

Since I was close enough to be the catalyst to this potentially traumatic event, I couldn't help but overhear the mother's reaction, as she spun and lowered herself to the youngster's level.

"Wow, honey, you're amazing! You caught yourself so quickly! What strong arms you have! You are so athletic!"

Turning to her other daughter, she continued, "Did you see how quickly Jesse reacted? Isn't she wonderful? I am so blessed that I have two incredible daughters with so much talent and grace. What an amazing day this is! Tonight's meal will be a celebration of my children."

She brushed off Jesse's clothing, embraced both daughters (took Jesse's hand), and the threesome disappeared into the eatery.

Aside from wanting to hug this prize-winning mother for instilling such fantastic and life-affirming attitudes, my initial reaction was a reminder of the power of words.

How often have we been unwitting victim, forced to endure over-hearing the painful tirade of a parent with lesser skills berating a youngster for a mistake? My soul cries for that child's future; it is bleak.

Yet, equally true — and infinitely more optimistic — is the empowered and unlimited tomorrows to be enjoyed by these sisters upon reaching womanhood. It is as assured as the fact that Jesse loves purple ponies.

What we say matters more than we realize. It affects what we feel, which determines what we do; in effect, carving out — word by word — the path of our lives. Not only is it vital what we say to our children, and to each other, but also equally as critical what we verbalize to ourselves.

When was the last time you referred to yourself as "amazing?" Jesse would tell you that you are.

OF ACNE AND PANT SIZES

I am reminded of my teen years.

One of the most tortuous events of adolescence is the explosion of pimples on one's facial landscape. Unbeknownst to most, these bulbous, bloated, bulging beacons of embarrassment have an intelligence of their own and connive to materialize at the worst possible moment — and in the most awful location. Therefore, it is guaranteed that the morning of the formal prom, one will be greeted in the mirror by a gargantuan red, inflamed, swollen one-inch zit on the tip of your nose. Take it to the bank.

Most people (yes, teens are people) are too polite to say anything when you appear to all the world like a caricature of W.C. Fields, any sinus commercial, and Bozo the Clown. Your day is spent inventing reasons why you cannot move your hand from the front of your face because even though you've tried to conceal the damage with two pounds of blemish makeup (causing your skin to develop the oh-so-attractive, tomblike cast of a mannequin), Captain Blackhead unflinchingly stands out front taunting, "Don't look him in the eyes; instead gawk intently at his red, puffy, swelling."

Ah, such special memories…

Acne might be a thing of my past, but the feelings of embarrassment are identical to when I feel bloated from excess consumption.

My stomach becomes a radio station, broadcasting on all channels: "This is a test of the emergency mortification system; for the next 60 minutes, please don't look anywhere else. Glare unblinkingly at his immense, distended, belly while pointing in a mocking fashion. Should this have been a real emergency, you would have been instructed to add humiliating comments. This is only a test."

To compensate, I suck in my abdomen, causing the tonal range of my voice to increase one octave while adding a slightly breathy quality to my speech. (I rationalize this, believing others find it a sexy addition to my speech pattern.)

Of course, there are problems with this approach, most notably would be sitting or bending; as one can never be sure of the tensile strength of button thread under strain. I would feel terrible should the round fastener explode forth from my midline, fly across the room, and put out somebody's eye. I wager the medical report would make history: "Blindness induced by excessive chocolate intake from out-of-control dieter in nearby restaurant booth."

Oh sure, I try using denial. When asked my pants size, I reply proudly (while loosening my belt), "32 W-L-D." Women have descriptors like "petite" or "junior;" why can't men?

"W-L-D? What's that?"

"While lying down." (Unfortunately, it's still a 36 when I stand up.)

The hottest fashion

Tumult is parading on the fashion catwalk.

According to Reuters, the world's first ban on overly thin models at a top-level fashion show has been announced in Madrid and is causing no small amount of concern within that industry. Underweight models (those with a body mass index — BMI — of under 18) will not be allowed to walk the runway. The reason cited by organizers is they "want to project an image of beauty and health, rather than waif-like or heroin chic." They believe (and they are most likely accurate) that young girls and women were trying to copy their rail-thin looks and were therefore developing eating disorders. (For comparison, the average American woman is 5' 4" and weighs 140, a BMI of 24, which is considered in the normal range of 18-25. The average American model is 5' 11" and weighs 117 pounds, a BMI of 16.)

I am torn by the decision in Spain.

It is not because I follow the latest designer news nor the ups and downs of Tommy Hilfiger, Donna Karan, or Calvin Klein. Although I find self-image, public health, and the plague of excess weight to be of utmost importance, I also believe personal choice is essential.

Every waking moment of each day, we make choices, which have repercussions; the results become our lives. Without the ability to make such decisions, our learning curve is thwarted and future decisions are poorer, making it more difficult to achieve our potential. Wisdom comes of evaluating our choices.

Conversely, until we possess that good judgment, it is society's moral imperative to protect the innocent from predators who view them as fodder for personal gain.

It is a conundrum. Choice becomes wisdom, which fosters better choices. Yet until we possess such understanding, others must direct our choices, slowing the expansion of wisdom.

More important however is not the dimensions of the model as much as the message of the event. I understand the need to be desirous of a contemporary and fresh appearance (although it matters less as I age). However, imagine a routine where high profile models were judged not by the hang of their outfits as much as the completeness of their character and the fulfilling of their potential.

Picture a catwalk adorned with women — and men — of every age, shape, and size. Each struts proudly a sense of purpose, social consciousness, creativity, knowledge, and — of course — health. Others are drawn to these events by the desire to better themselves and those around them. The ultimate "super model" becomes self-actualization — a fashion that fits beautifully on any body.

DANIEL & BRANDON

Losing a great deal of weight is not about eating less; rather it's about changing priorities. So, it stands to reason that when I lost my weight, I rearranged my life. One of those adjustments was to spend more time in the presence of my children and less in front of the refrigerator.

Daniel Scott Marcus was born November 17, 1983. His brother, Brandon Leigh came to this planet July 31, 1986. Day and night, Daniel is the actor: rowdy, dramatic, and boisterous. He is extremely willing to express unyielding, resolute opinions (whether asked or not) to anyone. Brandon is pensive, moderated — and although equally talented — more inclined to observe and suggest. His goal is writer/director.

Next week, the book of our lives enters its newest chapter as we load beds, boxes, and bicycles on a truck; they have heard the siren call of Hollywood, one seeks its spotlight, his brother desires fulfillment behind the camera.

After a painful, drawn-out divorce, I became a single father of these two artistic, very intelligent (doesn't every dad say that?) young men, attempting to keep a handle on everything from homework to heartaches. Our "group of three" attended movies on Fridays, over time growing from "The Lion King" to "Saving Private Ryan." I attended countless school plays, always spouting kudos (which — at times — was a masterwork of diplomacy). We disagreed (loudly) about personal boundaries and curfews. And when I remarried, I had the two best best men stand at my side.

Our story is no different than millions of other families. Names change, languages vary, paths take different roads, but this history — this particular one — is MY family. Although always together, we will no longer share one roof, and I am having a surprisingly, difficult adjustment.

Who will tell me — to the dollar — the gross receipts of each Hollywood release? How will I know what's up with Dave Mathews or Barenaked Ladies? From whom can I sneak garlic chicken pizza slices?

If I worry hard enough, can I protect them while they live elsewhere?

Am I still "Dad" when the noise of my sons no longer rebounds from the walls of my house?

This is their time and I have tried to prepare them (and me), always instructing, "do what you love, the money will follow." Who would think they would actually listen to "Pops" and follow his advice? And why must they do it so far away? Would it be wrong if I told them I was kidding?

This will be an emotional week. I might seek comfort foods. Please be gentle if you catch me.

BY THE NUMBERS

When I was learning to count, yet knowledgeable enough with arithmetic to no longer rely on fingers and toes, I pictured the largest number I could imagine: One Hundred. Nothing could be as immense as One Hundred, the King of the numerical empire. Counting to One Hundred was the pinnacle of accomplishment.

This column is our 100th get-together and, despite my increased counting skills, that number still carries significance. For two years, we have discussed health, diets, setbacks, and successes. (OK, actually I discussed it. But I always think of you when I write so that should count for something.)

To me, this is a milestone, a number with emotional significance. In achieving it, I realized how intricately, inextricably, woven into our lives are numbers.

My age? Number 52. Some get embarrassed about the number of years on the planet; I do not, as getting older beats its alternative. My wife and I have been married 6 years, together more than 12. These integers are a reflection of our commitment to each other. I have 2 sons. They live 700 miles away. I like the first number, not so much the second; I would prefer it to be lower. Nonetheless, numbers are what they are, unemotional reflections of the facts of our lives.

So, what's the deal with weight?

Before losing weight, there was no way I would not put "250" on my drivers license. Instead, I opted for a more ego-friendly number, 149, using the mentality of retailers who list prices ending in "9" to lull us into believing it's less costly. I don't fall for that tactic when I buy a sweater; I'm sure the DMV attendant didn't accept it when she saw my immense size. However, good public servant that she was, she let it pass. When my license arrived in the mailbox, sure enough, it showed me as an acceptable 149. Should occasion arise for me to weigh in somewhere — for example, the doctor's office — and the scale should say "250," I could snap out this legally binding document and have it corrected.

Funny how life works…

After losing my weight, and actually weighing 179, I renewed my license, eagerly listing — for the first time — the correct number of pounds. I proudly walked to the counter, handed in the application, gave her my old license, and waited while she did perused the poundage on my paperwork.

She analyzed my old license; studied my renewal, peered at me over the Ben Franklin spectacles perched on her nose, and stated, "179, huh? Last time, you only weighed 149. Might want to consider a diet."

SAVORING THE MOMENT

Some moments shoot by too swiftly. Instead of scurrying past, I wish they would linger, slowly, softly, simmering, allowing me to relish the warm richness of life's flavors.

I would cease time when my children first ventured forth uncertainly; wobbling on chubby infant legs, taking their first steps, the realization dawning that their world had just expanded. If that moment lived forever, I would harbor no regrets.

When I fell in love, realizing — this time — I had found my life partner, is another tick of the clock I would solidify. Right then, I felt a connection with an essence holy, ageless, and romantic. If Father Time froze me there, I would not complain.

Those moments, in which we languish, lazily and luxuriously, arrive without notice. Not all are life-changing benchmarks, reserved only for outstanding occasions. They are more frequent, oft times overlooked, as we hasten to get "where we're going," discounting where we are.

The arc of a rainbow across a dreary grey sky, brilliant colors patterned alongside a limitless and grand backdrop deserves a slowdown.

Arising on Saturday — covered neck to toes in a thick, fluffy, fresh comforter — with nothing on one's to-do list, and awakening to the plink-plop-plap of rain-drops against the window merits a slower pace. It is further enhanced when one's first thought — "Yich, it's Monday" — is replaced with the realization that rather, this morning is the first day of a lazy weekend.

Joyfully being infected by the uninhibited giggles of small children engaged in a magical world untouched by adult concerns is truly one of life's greatest pleasures. Why would anyone rush that?

Moments as those are common when one watches for them: a warm short-sleeve day on the boardwalk, a light breeze tussling your hair; the close-pressed hug of a friend as she greets you by chance in the course of daily tasks; a shared unexpected chuckle with the sales clerk behind the counter as you exchange pleasantries. They abound, invisible unless sought, adding spice and richness to our existence, making time on this planet worthwhile.

They also serve as reminders that not everything is to be hurried; some experiences need more time.

Always in such a helter-skelter, hell-bent, head-down hurry to lose my extra weight, I plead guilty to not paying attention to the blessings this process brings. Ignoring the confidence of a healthier body, dismissing the new found flexibility, pooh-poohing the confidence of my accomplishments; I am in such a sprint to get "there" that I take no pleasure from "here."

Some things take time. Some deserve it. This process is both.

BEWARE
AFTER-HALLOWEEN SALES

Tread wearily fellow dieter; the dark forces have gathered. Faster than a chocolate bat escaping the flames of Hades; quicker than a skeleton-costumed, sugar-crazed seven-year-old can consume a pile of gummi booty; we have arrived at the time of year when calories assail us from every direction.

One of the seemingly benign but more malevolent influences is the post-Halloween candy sale. Enter any store and be immediately accosted with an oversized display filled with foil covered peanut butter chocolate bats, black and orange jelly beans, and "fun size" candy bars. (Personally, I consider one-pound bars to be the "fun size" bars; miniatures are merely appetizers. But, who am I to quibble?) Attached to this colossal cache of calories is a sign proclaiming, "Half Off!"

Despite the activities of the previous evening, no amount of sugar crawling through my veins will cause me to pass up a 50% off sale; after all, I'm overweight, not stupid. Buy one, get one free, is a deal in which any rational person would partake. I therefore purchase four bags of high-fructose pleasure — saving five dollars — rationalizing it to the fact that I can freeze the treats for next year. I plan to use the five bucks for a low-calorie meal; truly, I have achieved a win-win scenario.

Despite noble intentions, too many marshmallow peanut bars have melted my willpower, and the treats do not survive until next October; actually they don't even endure the trip home. As I debate whether or not to curtain the damage after 7,353 calories, the mantra of all disillusioned dieters haunts its way into my caramel-coated consciousness, "As long as I blew it, I might as well really blow it and start dieting tomorrow." Whether 'tis the dark side of candy corn talking or not, this idea makes sense at the moment and from then on, anything slow enough to get a fork into it becomes my prey. Before dawn, I have consumed more calories than there are zombies walking the streets on all Hallow's eve.

This continues well into the week; soon my stomach resembles the familiar shape of oversized jack o' lantern and my belt can no longer traverse my midline. In order to enjoy the simple pleasure of breathing, I am forced to buy three larger pairs of pants ($29 each), a new belt ($10), and a pullover, extra-large shirt to rid me of the danger of buttons popping from my mid-section and putting someone's eye out ($23). Including tax I'm now out $153!

Of course, I did save five dollars on half price candy, making my net expenditure $148 but that's still one scary after-Halloween sale.

A LUCKY MAN

There is a fable whereby God gives each person the option to rid himself of his most pressing difficulty. Everyone places his or her problems in the center of a circle. In turn, each then inspects the travails and challenges of the others, and chooses what he or she would prefer. As the fable goes, everyone opts for his own problem. Human nature is to always consider oneself less fortunate than others — until presented with reality.

Michael J. Fox considers himself to be a "lucky man." As I watched him on TV try to contain uncontrollable tremors and twitches inflicted by Parkinson's disease, I was astonished — and awed — to hear him describe himself as "fortunate." He admits he would not have opted for this disease; yet as long as it is his path, he feels it is a gift because he's able to help others.

Shall we compare? Fox describes Parkinson's as "a gift;" I complain when I have to say "no" to a second scoop of ice cream. Maybe rethinking my position is in order.

Since I was a young overweight lad, I cannot remember when I did not complain about having to watch what I eat. While other children gorged themselves on potato chips, soft drinks, and chocolate fudge bars, my mother filled me with nonfat milk, fruit, and grilled chicken.

As a small boy stomping his feet in the midst of a tantrum, I would rail against the wrongness of the universe. "It's not fair!" I yelled. "Richard and Nancy are going to get ice cream. I want to go too!"

In those early years, I could not know the pain my mother felt as she was compelled to hold back her son from the experience of his peers so he could learn much-needed healthier habits. Lovingly, she would reply, "You're right; it's not fair. But Richard and Nancy don't have to watch their weight. You need to eat more carefully than they do."

I grew resentful over time: wounded by the loneliness felt only by the unattractive, angry over diets that promised but never delivered, insulted and beaten down by boorish comments poking fun of my size. Why did God condemn me?

Michael J. Fox — with Parkinson's — considers his disease a gift. I have an outburst over having to eat low-fat cheese. I'm thinking I just might need to "get over myself."

I "suffer" from a disease of abundance. While half the planet's population goes without, I must cut back. I must count calories in a world one person out of two prays not to go to sleep hungry.

If we were to put my problem in the circle, I think I'd take it back.

CORRECTLY CHOSEN COOKIES

At the local coffee house-slash-bakery, father and toddler daughter enter. Taking a break from my warmed over cup o' Joe and perusal of the newspaper, I observe as the scene unfolds.

An enthusiastic explosion of energy, curls, and exuberant youthfulness (with assistance from Dad), she shoves against the heavy glass door, and tripping over not-yet-fully-coordinated feet, stumbles with breathless anticipation to the bakery display booth, eager to discover this day's doughy fortunes. Nose hard-pressed against the case, splayed fingers smearing glass, her thoughts are as transparent as the window. Will today's selection be the round yellow smiley-face cookie with chocolate-drop eyes and licorice smile or a big, gooey, drippy, jelly-donut? Alas, this day they both shall be relegated to bridesmaid, not bride; her sparkling eyes having locked upon a smiling purple dinosaur cutout cookie with yellow lemony balloon in its doughy paw.

Decisions of such significance require adult confirmation; she glances toward daddy. "That one?" he confirms.

A momentary flash of internal reflection crosses her complexion while she analyzes options, finger in her mouth to help the process. Head nodding enthusiastically, unable to remove her stare from the cookie, she says eagerly, "Yes, that one."

Feet now dangling from her over-sized chair, every bite is savored with unabashed joy. Life is as it should be when one has a purple dinosaur cookie on one's plate. Can any being fairly ask for more than that?

Although more jaded, and having consumed far more meals than this cute youngster with bluish icing now smeared across her chin, I confess that while I do not kick flopping feet with flighty, frantic, exhilaration at the possibility of a T-Rex cookie, I have trouble focusing on my dining companion if the prospect of tiramisu or baked Alaska will bring to a close my repast.

Oft times, I have slogged through diets that punish me with bland, tasteless, textures, resembling packing materials more than foodstuffs. If that is the secret to a longer lifespan, I'm not sure it's worth it.

Sacrifice does have value; it strengthens character and teaches patience. However, in all things, balance is key. Experience joy at mealtime. Simply share a few bites with a friend — especially if she'll kick her feet and giggle with glee. Besides, it improves the meal.

Something Light

When on vacation, I dress quicker than my wife, having less hair, and therefore less of a need to blow-dry it. With the extra time, I find myself waiting for her at the hotel restaurant.

"What will it be this morning?" asks the waitress.

Studying the menu, I am engaged in a fierce internal debate between "responsible" (fresh fruit), and "desirable" (hash browns, bacon, omelet, croissant). Adult overrules inner child and I order "something light," oatmeal.

Momentarily a bathtub-size basin arrives. Submerged in thick, rich, cream, smothered with a brown syrupy liquid of melted maple sugar, is my hot cereal. Realizing it's too late to ask for nonfat milk and sugar on the side, I reassure myself the faux pas won't harm my diet. Everyone knows unintended calories don't count; fat cells realize the error and disregard the weight gain.

The waitress places a platter of sugary condiments on the table before leaving. At first, I am inclined to resist them, but reevaluate. Maybe this is a local tradition; it would be rude to offend our hosts. Besides, I'm on vacation; it's almost an edict that one sample new foods while traveling.

Rationale safely locked in place; to others I must appear to be an alchemist developing a brew in a caldron. I put in butter, honey, cream, yogurt (three flavors), strawberry jam, grape jelly, raw sugar, and cashews. I would mix in yet more but I'm concerned the table will buckle under the weight of my "light snack." The embarrassment could put a damper on my day.

Sipping down the concoction, I refill the bowl with sugary additives each time it drops below the rim. After a few iterations, I'm unsure any original oatmeal remains but I continue to add more flavorings as the rainbow swirl of reds, yellows, purples, and browns has me on a full-tilt sugar buzz and rational thinking is no longer an option.

My wife arrives, sliding into the booth as I clean the remains of the bowl. The inclination to use my finger like a spatula and scrape the edges is overruled in favor of a more mature demeanor.

She looks at the plate, "You ate already? I thought we were going to have breakfast together?"

"It was nothing, just a small bowl of oatmeal to hold me over."

The eating season

Dangerous days for dedicated, disciplined, dieters have descended. We now thunder headlong into an unending haze of fudge mints, eggnog lattes, and walnut cranberry honey stuffing. Activity and exercise levels, formerly consisting of lengthy walks through the trees and afternoons of yard work, plummet to gluteus-maximizing extended sessions plopped on the couch, watching television — a pyramid of cold mashed potatoes and cranberry sauce ever at the ready on the overflowing coffee table.

Some believe the "eating season" (as it should formally be named) begins in late November. In fact, as reliably as the annual return of the swallows to Capistrano, it opens with the first sighting of holiday ornaments in greeting-card stores, a much-heralded occurrence starting earlier each year. One day I'm dedicated to following my program. Twenty-four hours hence, holiday angels and cute ceramic teddy bears hanging from twinkling window displays pronounce, "Cast your waist to the wind. The holidays are here. Diet in January."

The zenith of this landscape of nonstop in(di)gestion is Thanksgiving.

With platters of sumptuous food extending beyond the horizon, this is the single celebration forcing dieters to dress appropriately. Oh sure, "Don we now our gay apparel" applies to holiday finery on

Christmas; but Thanksgiving — being also a test of endurance — requires shrewd planning. In the same manner that one would not run a marathon in a sequin-covered ball gown, it would be folly to attempt Thanksgiving's feasting in street apparel.

The following advice is for professional eaters only; do not attempt without supervision.

Be meticulous about choosing expandable outfits for that day, preferably sans belt; soft, nonbinding, elastic is my preference. Sweat pants, over-sized shirts, and large loose dresses are prized. (I have even considered wearing a Hawaiian MuMu but it clashes with my shoes.) As practiced athletes, pace caloric intake, starting cautiously before noon, careful not to peak too early, lest three cold-turkey-mashed-potato sandwiches, and half a pecan pie go uneaten before bedtime.

Staying conscious with so much food is indeed a challenge.

Yet, seriously, do remember that millions sleep on empty stomachs. Our unrelenting nag of dieting could be portrayed as a "curse of prosperity." While too many starve, we are so fortunate — so our concern is learning to consume less.

Stay aware about much you eat on Thanksgiving. Be thankful that you must.

OBESITY PILLS
AND STONE SOUP

May I have the envelope please? The winner of the "no-brainer" award goes to... (drum roll)... the National Institutes of Health!

I promise I'm not making this up: In a study by NIH that appeared in the New England Journal of Medicine, we discover that obese patients lose more weight if they make a lifestyle change in addition to taking a diet pill. Apparently, those who merely took medication and continued unchanged their "standard" routine lost only 11 pounds per year. Others, who swallowed the same medicine, but limited daily caloric intake to 1500, exercised, tracked their food, and attended a group; lost 27 pounds.

Please excuse me while I climb upon my soapbox.

Hello?!? This report is news? It goes without saying (or so I naively thought) that if one restricts calories, walks regularly, tracks eating habits, and elicits support; the unavoidable result will be fewer pounds. Frankly, I'm astonished it was only 27.

It brings to mind the "stone soup" fable. Entering a village with nothing to his name but a rock, a poverty-stricken vagabond seeking a meal discloses that he has an extraordinary stone. When boiled with water, it is the only ingredient necessary to bring forth a delicious soup. "Of course," he adds, "it will be better if the community would provide broth, vegetables, and other provisions." The population does so; the result is a rich, magnificent stew.

Naturally it was not the rock that made the flavor; everything else did. Equally obvious to me is the diet pill didn't cause the weight loss; everything else did.

Expecting to merely swallow a capsule and lose weight is tantamount to slipping into new tennis shoes, anticipating they provide the ability to run a marathon. Herbs, capsules, and tablets might be tools; but they are certainly not magic wands.

It is human to long for a supernatural concoction, which — without effort — provides youth, vigor, a flat belly, and the ability to rebuke both common sense and the laws of nutrition.

Bad news: it doesn't exist. And I agree; it's a full-size, colossal, cranky, bummer.

The good news is we're each capable and smart enough to succeed anyhow.

Yet, if you really believe a pill is all it takes to get skinny, there are folks who will try to sell you a bridge in San Francisco.

More times than not

Over several strong, black, cups of steaming coffee, we thrashed out matters of vital import. We agreed that if we ruled the world, it would operate quite differently; we were of one mind that aging enhances our best relationships. Then, came the mother of all questions: "How does one determine if ours was a 'Good Life' when time's up?"

That is probably a conclusion left to one infinitely wiser than two middle-aged mortals. Nonetheless, by unanimous consent, we established that if — in those final moments — the "ups" count higher than the "downs," the "happys" are more numerous than the "sads," indeed Life was good. In simple parlance, it's a "more-times-than-not thing," not a "100% thing."

Merely speculation, I am quick to admit; albeit it brings to me a sense of peace in present days. Oh yes, we also pledged that whomever gets to the other side first informs the other if we're correct. (And, dear reader — because I like you — I promise to publish it here if possible.)

Scene change: fast forward to present time.

I find myself – yet again – having to "get my act together" to repair damage I inflicted on my weight loss goals.

Throughout the entirety of Thanksgiving Day, I held myself back from cold turkey, mayonnaise sandwiches and manhole size servings of pumpkin pie. I was noble.

The day after? Well, that's a different story.

It began, as always, with a nibble here, a bite there. Not being a middle-of-the-road kind of guy however, I quickly reach a point where I decide, "as long as I blew it, I might as well REALLY blow it," and jump headlong over the cliff. History ignored is history repeated; here I stand again. You'd think after five decades, I'd have this figured out.

Yet… maybe I have.

If the key to a good life is "more-times-than-not," it stands to reason that success is "more-forward-than-backward." Peering though too constricted a window of time, perspective is distorted, all one sees is flaws and failures. Stepping back, a more accurate image comes into focus: habit change is indeed a "more-times-than-not thing," not a "100% thing." It is, after all, a fragment of Life.

It was a rough day, and I did set myself back. Today, however, has been great. I'm moving forward again.

You know, I just might yet get there.

RUTH

As she crossed the airport tarmac her hazel eyes found me, brilliant dancing lights of love; her cane and a jumbo purse (over-stuffed with low-calorie treats) dangled from an outstretched arm, her hands already reaching out to touch my face. No matter my age, life was better when Mom was in town.

She found it unthinkable to arrive without groceries. Upon entering my house, we would unload the luggage and put away the small food store she managed to cram into her carry-on.

"I brought grapefruit," she would begin without fail, pulling a half-dozen incredulously oversized, yellow, citrus globes from her carrier, "I know you're watching your weight; I wanted you to have something you could eat."

"I don't like grapefruit Mom."

"You don't?" Each and every time I reminded her she was surprised anew. "Since when don't you like grapefruit?"

"I have NEVER liked grapefruit."

"Really? Your sister likes grapefruit."

"I know Mom. We go through this every time you visit."

Oh, how I miss that dance.

While I went about my daily duties, she filed, cleaned and — like clockwork — read her ever-present dog-eared paperback. Of course, she also prepared meals — lots and lots of meals.

The kitchen table, obscured by an assortment of low calorie, high fiber, semi-tasteless pastries imported via suitcase, became a testing ground to sample new fare.

"Try this," she said, referencing a brown, crusty, splotch topped with a dollop of brick-red ooze, "only 80 calories, no sugar."

Normally, I would have steered clear, not trusting the food's appearance enough to smell it, let alone ingest it. But if Mom said do it, I would leap from cliffs; my welfare was her highest priority.

We lunched on tuna salads (made with no fat mayo between two slices of high fiber bread), fruit salads (with low-fat yogurt), and coffee. Hers — half regular, half decaffeinated — was incomplete without nonfat milk; it being so vital that she carried small plastic vials of it next to the pink sweetener packages in her purse.

Supportive and forever proud of me, she was a driving force in giving me the strength to lose weight.

This day would have been Ruth Marcus's 80th birthday. In a season of blessings, I felt you needed to know her.

THE NIGHT BEFORE CHRISTMAS

(with apologies to Clement Clarke Moore)

'Twas the night before Christmas
And all though my kitchen
Was cuisine of all kinds
Quite a bit — not a smidgen

The counter was covered with
Pies, turkey, and ham
And up on the stovetop
Ten pounds candied yams

Near a huge chocolate Santa
Lay Hanukkah gelt
Treats for my Jewish friends
'twould be appreciated, I felt

Eggnog in glasses
Filled with spiced rum
I downed several cupfuls
My downfall's begun

Cookies and nut rolls
And cakes of all kinds
I thought of my diet
But paid it no mind

Like a shopper after Christmas
I'm off on a mission
To rid future temptation
I'd empty the kitchen

First came the carving
Of drumstick and thigh
Giant mounds of potatoes
Next piled quite high

I downed a whole bird
The seasoning and such
And turned toward the casseroles
"That's really not much."

First a scoop, then a ladle
A bowl, and then four
I inhaled them quickly
And went back for more

On the table were sauces
And dressings made of nut
At the instant I ate them
Came pressure in my gut

So I paused for a moment
I needed some air
So much more to savor
This doesn't seem fair

I thought about stopping
These holiday dishes
Brown gravies, white sauces
They're just so delicious

My belt it was stretching
My pants were too tight
But leaving these goodies
Was certainly not right

Just one more small taste
And then off to bed
When then I did spy
Cookies - part green and part red

Star-shaped and snowflakes
All covered with sweet
A great way to finish
After twelve pounds of meat

I reached for the cookies
To put more food in
When suddenly I saw him
Dressed in red, with a grin

"Ho! Ho! Ho!" came his bellow
Then he saw what I ate
Every pan now was empty
And so were the plates

My stomach was bulging
My pants set to split
I felt really awful
Whether I stand or I sit

I wanted to be friendly
But couldn't make a sound
I needed full focus
Just to hold it all down

He stared quite intently
His smile, it was tacit
And said, "Here's your gift"
Eight gallons of antacid

GOOD PEOPLE

The airline and I differ on the concept of "completion." Please don't misunderstand; I certainly do not want the pilot attempting to land in pea-soup fog, as I have a passionate interest in my safe arrival. Yet, depositing me 150 miles from my destination (while still billing me for my ticket), and informing me, "You're on your own," is somewhat less than my idea of stellar service.

If not for the humanity of a warm-hearted dentist (and his wife) who drove a combined eight hours, I could be writing this while still in the Redding Municipal Airport. To those two rescuing angels, "Thank you; you're a blessing."

There are loads of good people, although sometimes it seems difficult to locate them. However, that which I seek, I usually find.

This begs a philosophical question: Are we basically self-absorbed, egocentric, insensitive beings forced into mutual cooperation solely out of legal requirements — or is it our nature to nurture and to support and care for others? Do we just get so wrapped up in our own life that we forget we share it?

In hopeful moments, I am convinced of the latter. My evidence is — despite glaring exceptions — when the trappings of civilization collapse, we revert to our basic natures. In those times, strangers assist strangers; community good is no longer enforced by edict, yet it blossoms.

In a very minor way, that's quite commonplace: An unfamiliar person holds open a heavy glass door to let you into the bakery. Someone unknown waves you into the long line of traffic on Broadway when leaving the parking lot. After spilling your purse at the grocery store, a young man chases you to return the five-dollar-bill you dropped.

Small deeds, yes, but so (under) appreciated.

Sometimes, I merely forget to look, and those hours become my darkest and most dreary. Feeling isolated, I seek comfort — so I eat. It makes little sense; nonetheless it is what I do.

At the dawn of a new year, when all things are still possible, might it be an appropriate moment to commit to seeking the light in each other? It may not help with dieting — but it definitely won't make it more difficult.

Be assured there are many first-rate people; smile at the one in the mirror.

Peace to all next year, beginning from within.

In two years

This is my 104th weekly column: two years. I am humbled and honored by the fact that you have helped me reach this landmark. It is the way that with milestones, come reflections.

I am not whom I was upon the commencement of this journey; I view the world in a different way. Although always curious, I am now more observant and analytical. I do not watch, I witness; seeking clarification, striving to make sense, always on alert for sparks of understanding and illumination that I can share via these pages. It is a way of connecting. It is also an educational, fascinating, enjoyable — albeit sometimes difficult — process. I rarely regret it.

Experience has led me to believe that the speed at which time passes is more perception than reality. We disappoint and set ourselves up to fail upon forgetting this vital lesson: Time accelerates when we enjoy its process; it lags when we struggle. In reality, time is what time is. How we feel about what we do adjusts the perceived speed of its passage.

When I was brand new, each morning was a fresh miracle cast in a yellow-orange hue. When I was that young, two years was forever. It was painful to count the days between vacations or holidays. To realize that I had to wait even a week to go to a birthday party was excruciating. Time crawled. The clock dragged. Because youthful energy made me eager to "get on with it," I struggled with the pace of life, and consequently, it jammed in slow motion.

It is human nature to want more, or to desire something better. Improved health, more understanding, increased prosperity — we know we will not "get there" in a day. There are a great many lessons to be learned. But because we so crave what we don't have, acquiring it seems to "take forever." We struggle and lament the process. In effect, we "slow down" the time it takes to be there. On the other hand, focusing on the joys of the lesson, the excitement of new knowledge, and the pride of accomplishment, causes time to flow without a hitch.

There is no small amount of irony here. Those things I want to do and enjoy go by in a blink. Chores and lessons won't get past me fast enough. Alas, accepting life on its own terms is yet another key to contentment.

I do know because I enjoy life, that "two years from now" will feel like it has arrived tomorrow. The previous two whooshed by at light speed, leaving me unsure they were even here.

Whatever I want to do next must begin immediately, as tomorrow is almost past.